AF443555

New Targets in Inflammation

Inhibitors of COX-2 or Adhesion Molecules

The publishers are grateful to
Dr Michelle Browner,
Roche Bioscience, Palo Alto, California,
for the schematic diagram of the
human COX-2 dimer shown on the cover

New Targets in Inflammation
Inhibitors of COX-2 or Adhesion Molecules

Edited by

DR NICOLAS BAZAN*, DR JACK BOTTING and SIR JOHN VANE
*The William Harvey Research Institute, Saint Bartholomew's Hospital
Medical College, London, United Kingdom
Neuroscience Center, Louisiana State University, New Orleans, USA

*Proceedings of a conference held on April 15–16, 1996,
in New Orleans, USA, supported by an educational grant from*

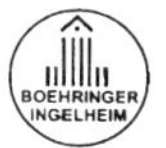

**Boehringer
Ingelheim**

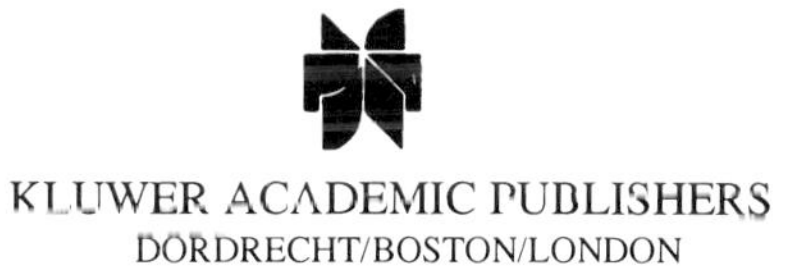

KLUWER ACADEMIC PUBLISHERS
DORDRECHT/BOSTON/LONDON

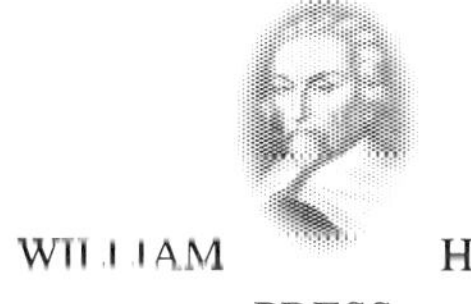

WILLIAM   HARVEY
PRESS

Distributors

for the United States and Canada: Kluwer Academic Publishers, PO Box 358, Accord Station,
Hingham, MA 02018-0358, USA
for all other countries: Kluwer Academic Publishers Group, Distribution Center, PO Box 322,
3300 AH Dordrecht, The Netherlands

A catalogue record for this book is available from the British Library

ISBN 0-7923-8714-7

Contents

List of Contributors

N. G. Bazan
LSU Neuroscience Center, Louisiana State University Medical Center, School of
Medicine, New Orleans, LA 70112, USA
Co-authors: V. M. Marcheselli, G. Allan, K. van Meter and J. P. Moises

W. Bolten
Rheumaklinik Wiesbaden II, Leibnizstrasse 23, 65191 Wiesbaden, Germany

M. Browner
Molecular Structure Department, Roche Bioscience, 3401 Hillview Avenue,
Palo Alto, CA 94303, USA

L. J. Crofford
Department of Internal Medicine, University of Michigan, 200 Zina Pitcher Place,
Ann Arbor, MI 48109-0531, USA

R. N. DuBois
Department of Medicine, Vanderbilt University Medical Center, Nashville,
TN 37232-2279, USA
Co-authors: A. Radhika, J. Shao, M. Tsujii, H. Sheng, O. Kobyashi,
R. D. Beauchamp and C. S. Williams

H. Fenner
Swiss Federal Institute of Technology, Zurich, Switzerland

S. H. Ferreira
Departamento de Farmacologia, Faculdade de Medicina de Ribeirão Preto, USP,
CEP 14.049-900, Ribeirão Preto, São Paulo, Brazil

A. W. Ford-Hutchinson
Merck Frosst Centre for Therapeutic Research, 16711 Trans Canada Highway,
Kirkland, Quebec II9H 3L1, Canada

G. A. Fitzgerald
The Center for Experimental Therapeutics, The University of Pennsylvania,
905 Stellar Chance Laboratories, 422 Curie Boulevard, Philadelphia, PA 19104, USA
Co-author: B. F. McAdam

H. Jick
Boston Collaborative Drug Surveillance Program, Boston University Medical
Center, 11 Muzzey Street, Lexington, MA 02173, USA

P. E. Lipsky
Harold C. Simmons Arthritis Research Center, University of Texas Southwestern
Medical School, 5323 Harry Hines Boulevard, Dallas, TX 75235-8884, USA
Co-authors: A. F. Kavanaugh, H. Schulze-Koops and L. S. Davis

P. J. Loll
Department of Pharmacology, University of Pennsylvania School of Medicine, 3620
Hamilton Walk, Philadelphia, PA 19104-6084, USA

S. Morham
Department of Pathology, University of North Carolina at Chapel Hill,
NC 27599-7525, USA
Co-author: R. Langenbach

M. Pairet
Department of Biological Research, Boehringer Ingelheim Research Laboratories,
Birkendorfer Strasse 65, 88397 Biberach an der Riss, Germany
Co-authors: L. Churchill and G. Engelhardt

J. R. Vane
The William Harvey Research Institute, St Bartholomew's Hospital Medical
College, Charterhouse Square, London EC1M 6BQ, UK
Co-author: R. M. Botting

P. A. Ward
Department of Pathology, University of Michigan Medical School,
1301 Catherine Road, Ann Arbor, MI 48109-0602, USA

Preface

For the past 100 years the mainstay of therapy for rheumatoid arthritis (RA) has been aspirin or other drugs of the non-steroid anti-inflammatory group. In 1971 Vane proposed that both the beneficial and toxic actions of these drugs was through inhibition of prostaglandin synthesis. The recent discovery that prostaglandins responsible for pain and other symptoms at inflammatory foci are synthesized by an inducible cyclooxygenase (COX-2) that is encoded by a gene distinct from that of the constitutive enzyme (COX-1) provided a new target for therapy of RA. A drug that would selectively inhibit COX-2 would hopefully produce the symptomatic benefit provided by existing NSAIDs without the gastrointestinal and renal toxicity due to the inhibition of COX-1. Drugs selective for COX-2 are now available. Experimental studies have shown them to be effective with minimal toxicity, and in clinical trials gastric and renal toxicities are less. Highly selective COX-2 inhibitors, perhaps designed with knowledge of the crystal structures of COX-1 and COX-2, are also available. Other experimental studies, including those in animals lacking effective genes for COX-1 or COX-2 and in experimental carcinomas, suggest there is still much to be learned of the pathophysiological functions of these enzymes.

The inflammatory response is a complex reaction involving many mediators that derive from white blood cells, endothelial cells and other tissues. Preliminary data have revealed that inhibitors of the cytokines and adhesion molecules that play a crucial role in the migration of white cells to inflammatory sites may be useful in RA. These various issues are reviewed by experts who have contributed the following chapters. Clearly such work will provide the basis for greatly improved treatments or even cures for inflammatory disease.

Nicolas G. Bazan
Jack H. Botting
John R. Vane

1 The history of anti-inflammatory drugs and their mechanism of action

J. R. VANE and R. M. BOTTING

The history of the anti-inflammatory drugs begins with the early use of decoctions or preparations of plants containing salicylate. Salicylic acid and salicylates are constituents of several plants long used as medicaments. About 3500 years ago the Egyptian Ebers papyrus recommended the application of a decoction of the dried leaves of myrtle to the abdomen and back to expel rheumatic pains from the womb. A thousand years later Hippocrates recommended the juices of the poplar tree for treating eye diseases and those of willow bark to relieve the pain of childbirth and to reduce fever. All of these medicinal remedies contain salicylates.

In AD 30 Celsus described the four classic signs of inflammation (rubor, calor, dolor and tumor; or redness, heat, pain and swelling) and used extracts of willow leaves to relieve them. Throughout the Roman times of Pliny the Elder, Dioscorides and Galen the use of salicylate-containing plants was further developed and willow bark was recommended for mild to moderate pain. In China and other parts of Asia also, salicylate-containing plants were being applied therapeutically. The curative effects of *Salix* and *Spiræa* species were also known to the early inhabitants of North America and South Africa.

Through the Middle Ages further uses for salicylates were found, such as plasters to treat wounds and various other external and internal applications, including the treatment of menstrual pain and discomfort of dysentery. However, willows were needed for basket making so the women herbalists of those days turned to other related plants: they grew meadowsweet (*Spiræa ulmaria*) in their herb gardens and made decoctions from the flowers.

The first 'clinical trial' of willow bark to be published in England was made by a country parson, the Reverend Edward Stone of Chipping Norton in Oxfordshire[1]. On June 2, 1763, Edward Stone presented a report to the Royal Society on the use of willow bark in fever. He had accidentally tasted it and was surprised by its extraordinary bitterness, which reminded him of the taste of cinchona bark (containing quinine), then being used to treat malaria. He believed in the 'doctrine of signatures' which dictated that the cures for diseases would be found in the same locations where the malady occurs. Since the "willow delights in a moist and wet soil, where agues chiefly abound", he gathered a pound of willow bark, dried it over a baker's oven for three months then ground it to a powder. His greatest success was with doses of 1 dram (1.8 g), which he reported using in about 50 patients with safety and success. He concluded his paper by saying "I have no other motives for publishing this valuable specific, than that it may have a fair and full trial in all its variety of circumstances and situations, and that the world may reap the benefits accruing from it". His wishes have certainly been realized; world production of aspirin has been estimated at 36 thousand tons a year, with an average consumption of about 70 tablets per person per year. Without the discovery in recent years of a great many replacements for aspirin and its variants, consumption would have surely been very much higher.

Salicylic acid was synthesized in Germany in 1860, and its ready supply led to even more extended usage as an external antiseptic, as an antipyretic and in the treatment of rheumatism. The father of Felix Hoffman, a young chemist working for Bayer, urged his son to make a more palatable form of salicylate to treat his severe rheumatism. Felix made acetylsalicylate or aspirin and asked his father to try it. Bayer's Research Director, Dr Heinrich Dreser, recognized that he had an important new drug on his hands and introduced it in 1899, at the same time writing a paper suggesting that aspirin was a convenient way of supplying the body with the active substance salicylate[2]. This point is still debated, but most of the evidence now shows that aspirin works in its own right.

By the early 1900s, the main therapeutic actions of aspirin (and sodium salicylate itself) were recognized as the antipyretic, anti-inflammatory and analgesic effects. With the passing of time several other drugs were discovered which shared some or all of these actions; these drugs include antipyrine, phenacetin, acetaminophen (paracetamol), phenylbutazone and, more recently, the fenamates, indomethacin and naproxen. Because of the similarity of their therapeutic actions these drugs tended to be regarded as a group and were generally known as the aspirin-like drugs. Because they were clearly distinct from the glucocorticoids (the other major group of agents used in the treatment of inflammation) these drugs were also referred to as non-steroid anti-inflammatory drugs (NSAIDs)[3].

Despite the diversity of their chemical structures, these drugs all share to some extent the same therapeutic properties. In varying doses they alleviate the swelling, redness and pain of inflammation, reduce a general fever and cure a headache. More than that, they also share to a greater or lesser extent a number of similar side effects. Depending on dose, they can cause gastric upset, in high doses delay the birth process and in overdose may damage the kidney. A particularly interesting 'side effect', now known as a therapeutic action, is the anti-thrombotic effect.

When a chemically diverse group of drugs all share not only the same therapeutic qualities (which in themselves have not much connection with each other) but also the same side effects, it is fairly certain that the actions of those drugs are based on a single biochemical intervention. For many years pharmacologists and biochemists searched for such a common mode of action without finding a generally acceptable scientific explanation.

SOME EARLY EXPLANATIONS FOR THE ACTION OF SALICYLATES

Before 1971, little was known about the real mechanism of action of the aspirin-like drugs except that they produced an anti-inflammatory effect which was qualitatively and quantitatively different from that of the anti-inflammatory steroids. In addition, many biochemical effects of the aspirin-like drugs had been documented, and theories based upon these effects abandoned. It was observed, for example, that most of these drugs uncoupled oxidative phosphorylation[4] and that several salicylates inhibited dehydrogenase enzymes, especially those dependent upon pyridine nucleotides[5,6]. Some aminotransferases[7] and decarboxylases[8] were also inhibited, as were several key enzymes involved in protein and RNA biosynthesis[9]. All of these inhibitory actions were at some time invoked to explain the therapeutic action of aspirin. A problem with most of these ideas was that the concentration of the drugs required for enzyme inhibition was in excess (sometimes greatly in excess) of the concentrations typically found in the plasma after therapy, and there was invariably a lack of correlation between the ability of these drugs to inhibit a particular enzyme, and their activity as anti-inflammatory agents[10]. Perhaps the most serious impediment to acceptance of any of the above ideas, however, was the fact that their proponents could not provide a convincing reason why inhibition of any of these enzymes should produce anti-inflammatory, analgesic and antipyretic effects.

It was, of course, not only biochemists who wondered how these drugs acted: pharmacologists were also intensely interested in their mechanism of action and no one contributed more important observations to this literature in the 1960s than the British pharmacologist Harry Collier. Collier had termed aspirin an 'antidefensive' drug because of its ability to prevent the physiological defence mechanisms of pain, fever and inflammation from functioning normally[11,12]. Together with his group he made the important finding that guinea-pigs treated with aspirin were protected from the bronchoconstriction normally elicited in these animals by bradykinin[13], ATP[14] or SRS-A (slow-reacting substance of anaphylaxis, now identified as a mixture of leukotrienes)[15].

It was, however, not clear how the bronchoconstrictor response was inhibited by aspirin. Initially, Collier suggested that 'A-receptors' (which could be blocked by aspirin-like drugs) were involved in the spasmogenic response to these agents[16], but he later abandoned this concept and wrote instead that the drugs acted "rather by inhibiting some underlying cellular mechanism that takes part to different extents in different responses mediated by different endogenous substances."

SALICYLATES AND THE PROSTAGLANDIN SYSTEM

It was, then, against this background of knowledge that the investigation of aspirin's action was taken over by researchers working with prostaglandins (PG). Priscilla Piper had been working with Harry Collier at the Parke Davis laboratories in Hounslow, Middlesex and came to Vane's laboratory at the Royal College of Surgeons as a graduate student. Piper and Vane employed the technique of continuous bioassay using the cascade bioassay system[17] developed by Vane in the mid 1960s for use with blood or an artificial salt solution. The method involved perfusing guinea pig isolated lungs with Krebs' solution and using the effluent to superfuse successively strips of vascular or gastrointestinal tissues selected for their sensitivity to different substances.

Piper and Vane found, as expected, the release during anaphylaxis of histamine and

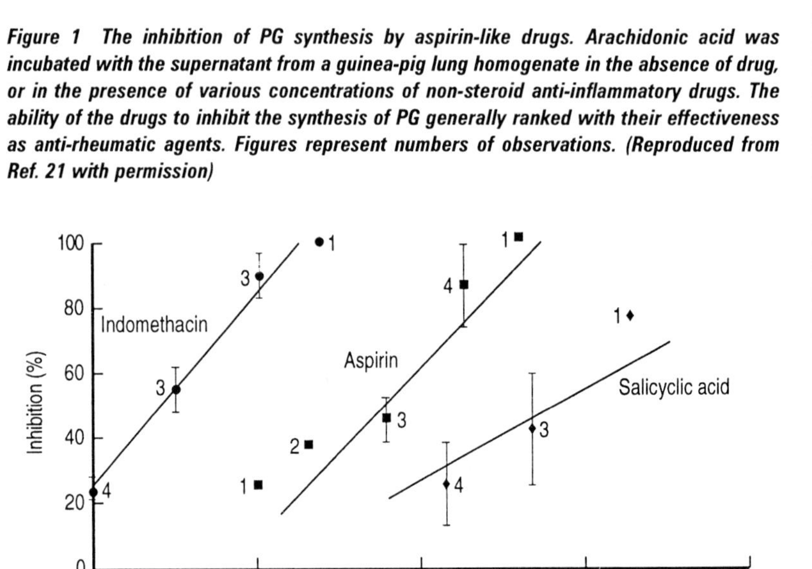

Figure 1 *The inhibition of PG synthesis by aspirin-like drugs. Arachidonic acid was incubated with the supernatant from a guinea-pig lung homogenate in the absence of drug, or in the presence of various concentrations of non-steroid anti-inflammatory drugs. The ability of the drugs to inhibit the synthesis of PG generally ranked with their effectiveness as anti-rheumatic agents. Figures represent numbers of observations. (Reproduced from Ref. 21 with permission)*

SRS-A but they also found some previously unreported substances: PG (mainly PGE_2 but with some $PGF_{2\alpha}$)[18] and another, very ephemeral, substance that, from the assay tissue that detected it, was called 'rabbit aorta contracting substance' (RCS). In the lung perfusate RCS had a half life of about 2 min and it was identified in 1975 as thromboxane A_2 (TXA_2) by Samuelsson's group[19]. It was RCS that provided the first clue to the relationship between aspirin and the PGs when Piper and Vane presented experimental evidence that the release of RCS from guinea pig isolated lungs during anaphylaxis was blocked by aspirin[20]. Indeed, almost any type of chemical or mechanical stimulus released both RCS and PGs. The result of these experiments was to move Vane's attention from RCS to PGs and he postulated that the various stimuli which released PGs were in fact 'turning on' the synthesis of these compounds. A logical corollary was that aspirin might well be blocking their synthesis.

He tested this idea using the supernatant of a broken cell homogenate from guinea pig lung as a source of PG synthase. There was a dose-dependent inhibition of PG formation by aspirin, salicylate and indomethacin but not by morphine[21]. Figure 1 shows the results of Vane's original experiment. Two other reports from the same laboratory in the same issue of *Nature* lent support to and extended his finding. Smith and Willis found that aspirin prevented the release of PG from aggregating human platelets[22] and Vane, Ferreira and Moncada demonstrated that aspirin-like drugs blocked PG release from the perfused, isolated spleen of the dog[23].

The discovery that each and every chemically diverse member of this large group of drugs all act by inhibiting cyclooxygenase (COX)[21] provided a unifying explanation of their therapeutic actions and firmly established certain PGs as important mediators of inflammatory disease (for reviews see Refs 24, 25, 26).

THE TWO COX ISOFORMS

A homogeneous, enzymatically active COX or PG endoperoxide synthase (PGHS) was isolated in 1976[27]. This membrane-bound haemo- and glycoprotein with a molecular weight of 71 kDa is found in greatest amounts in the endoplasmic reticulum of prostanoid-forming cells[28]. It exhibits COX activity which both cyclizes arachidonic acid and adds the 15-hydroperoxy group to form PGG_2. The hydroperoxy group of PGG_2 is reduced to the hydroxy group of PGH_2 by a peroxidase that utilizes a wide variety of compounds to provide the requisite pair of electrons. Both COX and hydroperoxidase activities are contained in the same dimeric protein molecule.

We now know that COX exists in at least two isoforms, COX-1 and COX-2. Over the last two decades, several new NSAIDs have reached the market based on enzyme screens which turned out to be against COX-1. Garavito and his colleagues[29] have determined the three dimensional structure of COX-1, providing a new understanding for the actions of COX inhibitors. This bifunctional enzyme comprises three independent folding units: an epidermal growth factor-like domain, a membrane-binding motif and an enzymatic domain. The sites for peroxidase and cyclooxygenase activity are adjacent but spatially distinct. The confirmation of the membrane-binding motif strongly suggests that the enzyme integrates into only a single leaflet of the lipid bilayer and is thus a monotopic membrane protein. Three of the helices of the structure form the entrance to the COX channel and their insertion into the membrane could allow arachidonic acid to gain access to the active site from the interior of the bilayer.

The COX active site is a long hydrophobic channel and Garavito et al.[29] present arguments that some of the aspirin-like drugs, such as flurbiprofen, inhibit COX-1 by excluding arachidonate from the upper portion of the channel. Tyrosine 385 and serine 530 are at the apex of the long active site. Aspirin irreversibly inhibits COX-1 by acetylation of the serine 530, thereby excluding access for arachidonic acid[30]. The S(–) stereoisomer of flurbiprofen interacts, via its carboxylate, with arginine 120, thereby placing the second phenyl ring within Van der Waal's contact of tyrosine 385. There may be a number of other sub-sites for drug binding in the narrow channel. The X-ray crystal structure of COX-2 closely resembles that of COX-1 and the binding sites for arachidonic acid on these enzymes are also very similar. Selectivity for inhibitors may be conferred by alternative conformations at the NSAIDs binding site in the COX channel.

PHYSIOLOGY OF COX-1 AND COX-2

The constitutive isoform of COX, COX-1, has clear physiological functions. Its activation leads, for instance, to the production of prostacyclin which when released by the endothelium is anti-thrombogenic[31] and when released by the gastric mucosa is cytoprotective[32]. The inducible isoform, COX-2, was discovered some 5 years ago and is induced in a number of cells by pro-inflammatory stimuli[33]. Its existence was first suspected when Needleman and his group reported that bacterial lipopolysaccharide increased the synthesis of prostaglandins in human monocytes in vitro[34] and in mouse peritoneal macrophages in vivo[35]. This increase was inhibited by dexamethasone and associated with de novo synthesis of new COX protein. A year or so later, an inducible COX was identified as a distinct isoform of cyclooxygenase (COX-2) encoded by a different gene from COX-1[36–39]. The amino acid sequence of its cDNA shows a 60% homology with the sequence of the non-inducible enzyme, with the size of the mRNA for the inducible enzyme approximating 4.5 kb and that of the constitutive enzyme being 2.8 kb. However, both enzymes have a molecular weight of 71 kDa and similar active sites for the natural substrate and for blockade by NSAIDs. The inhibition by the glucocorticoids of the expression of COX-2 is an additional aspect of the anti-inflammatory action of the corticosteroids. Levels of COX-2 are normally very low in cells and are tightly controlled by a number of factors including cytokines, intracellular messengers and the availability of substrate.

Since COX-2 is induced by inflammatory stimuli and by cytokines in migratory and other cells it is attractive to suggest that the anti-inflammatory actions of NSAIDs are due to the inhibition of COX-2, whereas the unwanted side effects such as irritation of the stomach lining and toxic effects on the kidney are due to inhibition of the constitutive enzyme, COX-1.

Over the years, the theory that inhibition of prostaglandin formation accounts for the therapeutic activity and the side effects of the aspirin-like drugs has been challenged, notably by Weissmann[40]. His arguments were partly based on comparing the actions of salicylate and aspirin, which are said to be equally effective against arthritis in the clinic[41], whereas in the original observations on COX[21] aspirin was 10 times stronger than salicylate as an inhibitor. As Weissmann's comparisons were based on COX-1, this apparent contradiction may now be explained by the existence of the two isoforms of COX, for salicylate and aspirin are both almost equally weak inhibitors of COX-2 although the mechanism of action of salicylate may be compounded by a suppression of the induction of COX[42].

Paracetamol also posed a problem for the original theory, for in therapeutic doses it has weak anti-inflammatory activity but is a stronger analgesic and antipyretic[43]. In 1972, we showed that COX preparations from the brain were more sensitive to paracetamol than those from the spleen and suggested that there may be different isoforms of COX[44]. Perhaps in the light of recent discoveries, there is also a COX-3 on which paracetamol has a preferential action.

PATHOPHYSIOLOGY OF COX-1 and COX-2

Several papers on COX-1 and COX-2 gene-deficient mice have now been published[45–47]. At first sight, some of the results are surprising until it is remembered that in both physiology and pathology the body uses several parallel pathways to reinforce a common result. For instance, it might have been expected that without the ability to generate prostacyclin, the gastric mucosa of COX-1 knockout mice would show the kind of erosions produced by NSAIDs. However, COX-1 (−/−) mice have normal gastric mucosa, albeit with a decreased sensitivity to the damaging effects of indomethacin[45]. The normality of the mucosa in these mice could well be brought about by the continued release of nitric oxide and CGRP, both also known to contribute to the maintenance of a healthy mucosa[48]. It is possible that in COX-1 (−/−) mice these mechanisms are accentuated to compensate for the lack of prostacyclin.

It is more difficult to explain the reduced ulcerogenic actions of indomethacin in these knockout mice. However, in concentrations higher than those needed to inhibit cyclooxygenase indomethacin inhibits many other enzyme systems. Furthermore, several aspirin-like drugs (including indomethacin) have a local irritant effect on the mucosa, as well as inhibiting COX through a systemic action[49]. Such a local irritation might explain the erosions in the COX-1 (−/−) mice, in which case subcutaneous indomethacin would have less effect.

In both COX-1[45] and COX-2 knockout mice[46,47] arachidonic acid applied locally still produces some ear inflammation. It should be noted that arachidonic acid leads not only to synthesis of COX products but also to leukotrienes via the 5-lipoxygenase pathway. Indeed, that the second pathway contributes to this inflammatory response is shown by 5-lipoxygenase knockout mice in which inflammation of the ear produced by arachidonic acid is substantially reduced[50]. When stronger and more general inflammatory stimuli are used (such as phorbol esters), many additional mediators will be called into play, including 5-hydroxytryptamine, bradykinin, nitric oxide and histamine. Thus, it is not surprising to a pharmacologist that cancelling out a single enzyme, such as COX-1[45], COX-2[46,47] or 5-lipoxygenase[50] has little or no effect on the gross inflammation induced by painting the ears with such a strong irritant as a phorbol ester.

Thus, the apparent paradox presented by studies in knockout mice may be logically explained. However, there are many relevant measurements still to be made in these gene-deficient strains of mice.

SELECTIVE INHIBITION OF COX-2

The importance of the discovery of inducible COX-2 is highlighted by the differences in pharmacology of the two enzymes[51]. Aspirin, indomethacin and ibuprofen are much less active against COX-2 than against COX-1[52]. Indeed, the strongest inhibitors of COX-1 such as aspirin, indomethacin and piroxicam are the NSAIDs which cause the most damage to the stomach[53]. The spectrum of activities of some ten standard NSAIDs against the two enzymes ranges from a high selectivity towards COX-1 (166-fold for aspirin) through to equiactivity on both[54].

The range of activities of NSAIDs against COX-1 compared with COX-2 explains the variations in the side effects exhibited by NSAIDs at their anti-inflammatory doses. Drugs which have the highest potency on COX-2 and a better COX-2/COX-1 activity ratio will have potent anti-inflammatory activity with fewer side effects on the stomach and kidney. Garcia Rodriguez and Jick[55] have published a comparison of epidemiological data on the side effects of NSAIDs. Piroxicam and indomethacin in

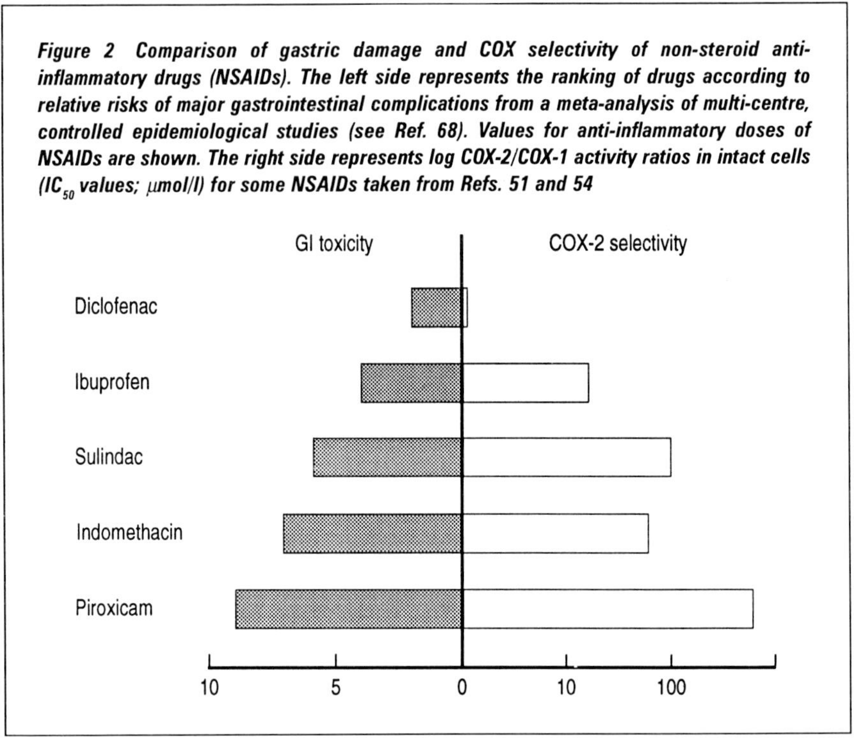

Figure 2   Comparison of gastric damage and COX selectivity of non-steroid anti-inflammatory drugs (NSAIDs). The left side represents the ranking of drugs according to relative risks of major gastrointestinal complications from a meta-analysis of multi-centre, controlled epidemiological studies (see Ref. 68). Values for anti-inflammatory doses of NSAIDs are shown. The right side represents log COX-2/COX-1 activity ratios in intact cells (IC$_{50}$ values; μmol/l) for some NSAIDs taken from Refs. 51 and 54

anti-inflammatory doses were found to produce high gastrointestinal toxicity: these drugs are much more potent against COX-1 than against COX-2[56]. Thus, when epidemiological results are compared with COX-2/COX-1 ratios, there is a parallel relationship between gastrointestinal side effects and COX-2/COX-1 ratios (Figure 2).

It should be noted that the COX-2/COX-1 ratio varies from test system to test system. For instance, reference 51, from which Figure 2 is taken, gives ratios for naproxen of 0.6 and for diclofenac of 0.7. However, using a microsomal enzyme preparation, Churchill et al.[60] found ratios of ~18.5 for naproxen and 0.5 for diclofenac.

Differences between systems are due to species or cell variations and possibly to length of incubation with the aspirin-like drug. Clearly, in correlating these ratios with the epidemiological and clinical data it must also be remembered that at anti-inflammatory doses both naproxen and diclofenac produce more severe gastric damage than meloxicam[67].

The discovery of COX-2 has stimulated several laboratories to develop selective inhibitors of this enzyme. Needleman and his group at Monsanto/Searle have made inhibitors which are some 1000-fold more potent against COX-2 than against COX-1[57]. One of these, SC-58635, is an effective analgesic for moderate to severe pain following tooth extraction[58]. A recent report described the selective COX-2 inhibitor from Merck-Frosst, L-475,337[59]. This compound was also 1000-fold more selective

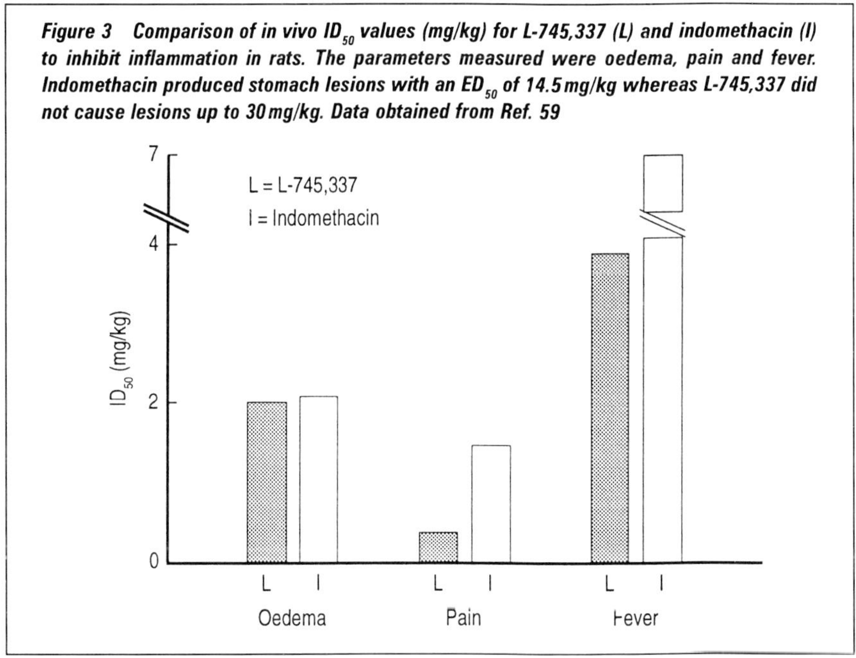

Figure 3   Comparison of in vivo ID_{50} values (mg/kg) for L-745,337 (L) and indomethacin (I) to inhibit inflammation in rats. The parameters measured were oedema, pain and fever. Indomethacin produced stomach lesions with an ED_{50} of 14.5 mg/kg whereas L-745,337 did not cause lesions up to 30 mg/kg. Data obtained from Ref. 59

for COX-2 in vitro with a good anti-inflammatory profile in animal models (Figure 3). Meloxicam is a new potent anti-inflammatory drug with selectivity as an inhibitor of COX-2. It has already been registered in several countries worldwide for use in patients with rheumatoid arthritis and osteoarthritis (Pairet, M.; see later this monograph). Using human recombinant enzymes in whole cells the ratio of IC_{50} values for COX-2 relative to COX-1 of meloxicam is 0.07, which demonstrates its selectivity in favour of COX-2[60]. DuP-697, flosulide (CGP 28238) and nimesulide were reported some years ago[61–63] to be potent anti-inflammatory drugs which did not cause stomach ulcers or alter renal blood flow. It is now clear that they are also selective inhibitors of COX-2. Nimesulide is on the market in Italy, Portugal and Greece as an anti-inflammatory analgesic despite a limited clinical profile. An effective selectivity for COX-2 was also shown for NS-398, made by the Taisho Pharmaceutical Company in Saitama, Japan[64]. However, selective COX-2 inhibitors may not be as potent as steroids, even though the lack of side effects will allow higher dosage. This is because PGs are not the only mediators involved in chronic inflammation. Nevertheless, arthritic patients will surely benefit before the year 2000 from the important discovery of more selective COX-2 inhibitors.

CONCLUSIONS

All the results so far published (and many yet to be published from the drug industry), support the hypothesis that the unwanted side effects of NSAIDs are due to their ability to inhibit COX-1 whilst their anti-inflammatory (therapeutic) effects are due to inhibition of COX-2. Other roles for COX-2 will surely be found in the next few years, for PG formation is under strong control in organs such as the uterus. It is likely that the hormonal induction of COX-2 leads to, for example, the PG production associated with parturition. The identification of selective inhibitors of COX-1 and COX-2 will not only provide an opportunity to test the new hypothesis but also lead to advances in the therapy of inflammation. New uses will also be found for selective COX-2 inhibitors. For example, aspirin is effective in the prophylaxis of colon cancer and we now know that it is COX-2 which is associated with this condition[65,66].

Acknowledgements

The William Harvey Research Institute is supported by grants from the Ono Pharmaceutical Company, Schwarz Pharma Limited and the Servier International Research Institute.

References

1. Stone E. An account of the success of the bark of the willow in the cure of agues. Phil Trans R Soc. 1763;53:195–200.
2. Dreser H. Pharmacologisches über Aspirin (Acetylsalicyl-saüre). Pflügers Arch. 1899;76:306–18.
3. Flower RJ. Drugs which inhibit prostaglandin biosynthesis. Pharmacol Rev. 1974;26:33–67.
4. Whitehouse MW, Haslam JM. Ability of some antirheumatic drugs to uncouple oxidative phosphorylation. Nature. 1962;196:1323–4.
5. Hines WJW, Smith MJH. Inhibition of dehydrogenases by salicylate. Nature. 1964;201:192.
6. Smith MJH, Bryant C, Hines WJW. Reversal by nicotinamide adenine dinucleotide of the inhibitory action of salicylate on mitochondrial malate dehydrogenase. Nature. 1964;202:96–7.
7. Gould BJ, Smith MJH. Salicylate and aminotransferases. J Pharm Pharmacol. 1965;17:83–8.
8. Gould BJ, Smith MJH. Inhibition of rat brain glutamate decarboxylase activity by salicylate in vitro. J Pharm Pharmacol. 1965;17:15–18.
9. Weiss WP, Campbell PL, Diebler GE, Sokoloff L. Effects of salicylate on amino acid incorporation into protein. J Pharmacol Exp Ther. 1962;136:366–71.
10. Whitehouse MW. Some biochemical and pharmacological properties of anti-inflammatory drugs. Prog Drug Res. 1965;8:321–429.
11. Collier HOJ. Aspirin. Sci Am. 1963;209:97–108.
12. Collier HOJ. A pharmacological analysis of aspirin. Adv Pharmacol Chemother. 1969;7:333–405.
13. Collier HOJ, Shorley PG. Analgesic antipyretic drugs as antagonists of bradykinin. Br J Pharmacol. 1960;15:601–10.
14. Collier HOJ, James GWL, Schneider C. Antagonism by aspirin and fenamates of broncho-constriction and nociception induced by adenosine-5'-triphosphate. Nature. 1966;212:411–12.
15. Berry PA, Collier HOJ. Bronchoconstrictor action and antagonism of a slow reacting substance from anaphylaxis of guinea-pig isolated lung. Br J Pharmacol. 1964;23:201–16.
16. Collier HOJ, Sweatman WJF. Antagonism by fenamates of prostaglandin $F_{2\alpha}$ and of slow reacting substance on human bronchial muscle. Nature. 1968;219:864–5.
17. Vane JR. The use of isolated organs for detecting active substances in the circulating blood. Br J Pharmacol Chemother. 1964;23:360–73.
18. Piper PJ, Vane JR. The release of prostaglandins during anaphylaxis in guinea-pig isolated lungs. In: Mantegazza P, Horton EW, editors. Prostaglandins, Peptides and Amines. London/New York: Academic Press, 1969:15–19.
19. Hamberg M, Svensson J, Samuelsson B. Thromboxanes: a new group of biologically active compounds derived from prostaglandin endoperoxides. Proc Natl Acad Sci USA. 1975;72:2994–8.

20. Palmer MA, Piper PJ, Vane JR. The release of RCS from chopped lung and its antagonism by anti-inflammatory drugs. Br J Pharmacol. 1970;40:581P
21. Vane JR. Inhibition of prostaglandin synthesis as a mechanism of action for aspirin-like drugs. Nature New Biol. 1971;231:232−5.
22. Smith JH, Willis AL. Aspirin selectively inhibits prostaglandin production in human platelets. Nature. 1971;231:235−7.
23. Ferreira SH, Moncada S, Vane JR. Indomethacin and aspirin abolish prostaglandin release from spleen. Nature. 1971;231:237−9.
24. Flower RJ, Vane JR. Inhibition of prostaglandin biosynthesis. Biochem Pharmacol. 1974; 23:1439−50.
25. Higgs GA, Moncada S, Vane JR. Eicosanoids in inflammation. Ann Clin Res. 1984;16:287−99.
26. Vane JR, Botting RM. The mode of action of anti-inflammatory drugs. Postgrad Med J. 1990; 66(Suppl.4):S2−S17.
27. Hemler M, Lands WEM, Smith WL. Purification of the cyclo-oxygenase that forms prostaglandins. Demonstration of the two forms of iron in the holoenzyme. J Biol Chem. 1976;251:5575−9.
28. Smith WL. Prostaglandin biosynthesis and its compartmentation in vascular smooth muscle and endothelial cells. Annu Rev Physiol. 1986;48:251−62.
29. Picot D, Loll PJ, Garavito RM. The X-ray crystal structure of the membrane protein prostaglandin H_2 synthase-1. Nature. 1994;367:243−9.
30. Roth GJ, Stanford N, Majerus PW. Acetylation of prostaglandin synthetase by aspirin. Proc Natl Acad Sci USA. 1975;72:3073−6.
31. Moncada S, Gryglewski R, Bunting S, Vane JR. An enzyme isolated from arteries transforms prostaglandin endoperoxides to an unstable substance that inhibits platelet aggregation. Nature. 1976;263:663−5.
32. Whittle BJR, Higgs GA, Eakins KE, Moncada S, Vane JR. Selective inhibition of prostaglandin production in inflammatory exudates and gastric mucosa. Nature. 1980;284:271 3.
33. Xie W, Robertson DL, Simmons DL. Mitogen-inducible prostaglandin G/H synthase: a new target for nonsteroidal antiinflammatory drugs. Drug Dev Res. 1992;25:249−65.
34. Fu J-Y, Masferrer JL, Seibert K, Raz A, Needleman P. The induction and suppression of prostaglandin H_2 synthase (cyclooxygenase) in human monocytes. J Biol Chem. 1990;265:16737−40.
35. Masferrer JL, Zweifel BS, Seibert K, Needleman P. Selective regulation of cellular cyclo-oxygenase by dexamethasone and endotoxin in mice. J Clin Invest. 1990;86:1375−9.
36. Xie W, Chipman JG, Robertson DL, Erikson RL, Simmons DL. Expression of a mitogen-responsive gene encoding prostaglandin synthase is regulated by mRNA splicing. Proc Natl Acad Sci USA. 1991;88:2692−6.
37. O'Banion MK, Sadowski HB, Winn V, Young DA. A serum- and glucocorticoid-regulated 4-kilobase mRNA encodes a cyclooxygenase-related protein. J Biol Chem. 1991;266:23261−7.
38. Kujubu DA, Fletcher BS, Varnum BC, Lim RW, Herschman HR. TIS10, a phorbol ester tumor promoter-inducible mRNA from Swiss 3T3 cells, encodes a novel prostaglandin synthase/cyclo-oxygenase homologue. J Biol Chem. 1991;266:12866−72.
39. Sirois J, Richards JS. Purification and characterisation of a novel, distinct isoform of prostaglandin endoperoxide synthase induced by human chorionic gonadotropin in granulosa cells of rat preovulatory follicles. J Biol Chem. 1992;267:6382−8.
40. Weissmann G. Prostaglandins as modulators rather than mediators of inflammation. J Lipid Med. 1993;6:275−86.
41. Weissmann G. Aspirin. Sci Am. 1991;January:84−90.
42. Wu KK, Sanduja R, Tsai AL, Ferhanoglu B, Loose-Mitchell DS. Aspirin inhibits interleukin-1-induced prostaglandin H synthase expression in cultured endothelial cells. Proc Natl Acad Sci USA. 1991;88:2384−7.
43. Clissold SP. Paracetamol and phenacetin. Drugs. 1986;32(Suppl. 4):46−59.
44. Flower RJ, Vane JR. Inhibition of prostaglandin synthetase in brain explains the antipyretic activity of paracetamol (4-acetamidophenol). Nature. 1972;240:410−11.
45. Langenbach R, Morham SG, Tiano HF et al. Prostaglandin synthase 1 gene disruption in mice reduces arachidonic acid-induced inflammation and indomethacin-induced gastric ulceration. Cell. 1995;83:483−92.
46. Morham SG, Langenbach R, Loftin CD et al. Prostaglandin synthase 2 gene disruption causes renal pathology in the mouse. Cell. 1995;83:473−82.

47. Dinchuck JE, Car BD, Focht RJ et al. Renal abnormalities and an altered inflammatory response in mice lacking cyclooxygenase II. Nature. 1995;378:406–9.

48. Whittle BJR. Neuronal and endothelium-derived mediators in the modulation of the gastric microcirculation: integrity in the balance. Br J Pharmacol. 1993;110:3–17.

49. Rainsford KD, Willis C. Relationship of gastric mucosal damage induced in pigs by anti-inflammatory drugs to their effects on prostaglandin production. Dig Dis Sci. 1982;27:624–35.

50. Chen XS, Sheller JR, Johnson EN, Funk CD. Role of leukotrienes revealed by targeted disruption of the 5-lipoxygenase gene. Nature. 1994;372:179–82.

51. Mitchell JA, Akarasereenont P, Thiemermann C, Flower RJ, Vane JR. Selectivity of nonsteroidal antiinflammatory drugs as inhibitors of constitutive and inducible cyclooxygenase. Proc Natl Acad Sci USA. 1993;90:11693–7.

52. Meade EA, Smith WL, DeWitt DL. Differential inhibition of prostaglandin endoperoxide synthase (cyclooxygenase) isozymes by aspirin and other non-steroidal anti-inflammatory drugs. J Biol Chem. 1993;268:6610–14

53. Lanza FL. A review of gastric ulcer and gastroduodenal injury in normal volunteers receiving aspirin and other non-steroidal anti-inflammatory drugs. Scand J Gastroenterol. 1989;24(Suppl. 163):24–31.

54. Akarasereenont P, Mitchell JA, Theimermann C, Vane JR. Relative potency of nonsteroid anti-inflammatory drugs as inhibitors of cyclooxygenase-1 or cyclooxygenase-2. Br J Pharmacol. 1994;112(Suppl.):183P.

55. Garcia Rodriguez LA, Jick H. Risk of upper gastrointestinal bleeding and perforation associated with individual non-steroidal anti-inflammatory drugs. Lancet. 1994;343:769–72.

56. Vane JR, Botting RM. New insights into the mode of action of anti-inflammatory drugs. Inflamm Res. 1995;44:1–10.

57. Isakson P, Seibert K, Masferrer J, Salvemini D, Lee L, Needleman P. Discovery of a better aspirin. Presented at the Ninth International Conference on Prostaglandins and Related Compounds. Florence, Italy, June 1994.

58. Hubbard RC, Mehlisch DR, Jasper DR, Nugent MJ, Yu S, Isakson PC. SC-58635, a highly selective inhibitor of COX-2, is an effective analgesic in an acute post-surgical pain model. J Invest Med. 1996;44:293A.

59. Chan C-C, Boyce S, Brideau C et al. Pharmacology of a selective cyclooxygenase-2 inhibitor, L-745,337: a novel nonsteroidal anti-inflammatory agent with an ulcerogenic sparing effect in rat and nonhuman primate stomach. J Pharmacol Exp Ther. 1995;274:1531–7.

60. Churchill L, Graham A, Shih C-K, Pauletti D, Farina PR, Grob PM. Selective inhibition of human cyclooxygenase-2 by meloxicam. Inflammopharmacology. 1996;4:125–35.

61. Gans KR, Galbraith W, Roman RJ et al. Anti-inflammatory and safety profile of DuP 697, a novel orally effective prostaglandin synthesis inhibitor. J Pharmacol Exp Ther. 1990;254:180–7.

62. Böttcher I, Schweizer A, Glatt M, Werner H. A sulphonamidoindanone CGP 28237 (ZK 34228), a novel non-steroidal anti-inflammatory agent without gastrointestinal ulcerogenicity in rats. Drugs Exp Clin Res. 1987;13:237–45.

63. Carr DP, Henn R, Green JR, Böttcher I. Comparison of the systemic inhibition of thromboxane synthesis, anti-inflammatory activity and gastro-intestinal toxicity of non-steroidal anti-inflammatory drugs in the rat. Agents Actions. 1986;19:374–5.

64. Futaki N, Takahashi S, Yokoyama M, Arai S, Higuchi S, Otomo S. NS-398, a new anti-inflammatory agent, selectively inhibits prostaglandin G/H synthase/cyclooxygenase (COX-2) activity in vitro. Prostaglandins. 1994;47:55–9.

65. Thun MJ, Namboodiri MM, Heath CWJ. Aspirin use and reduced risk of fatal colon cancer. N Engl J Med. 1991;325:1593–6.

66. Eberhart CE, Coffey RJ, Radhika A, Giardiello FM, Ferrenbach S, DuBois RN. Up-regulation of cyclooxygenase 2 gene expression in human colorectal adenomas and adenocarcinomas. Gastroenterology. 1994;104:1183–8.

67. Distel M, Mueller C, Bluhmki E, Fries J. Safety of meloxicam: a global analysis of clinical trials. Br J Rheumatol. 1996;35(Suppl. 1):68–77.

68. Henry D, Lim LL-Y, Rodriguez LAG et al. Variability in risk of gastrointestinal complications with individual non-steroidal anti-inflammatory drugs: results of a collaborative meta-analysis. Br Med J. 1996;312:1563–6.

2 Structure of prostaglandin H₂ synthase-1 (COX-1) and its NSAID binding sites

P. J. LOLL

Prostaglandin H_2 synthase (PGHS; also known as cyclooxygenase, COX) catalyses the first committed step in the conversion of arachidonic acid to prostaglandins (PG) and thromboxanes[1]. PGHS has two distinct enzymatic activities: a cyclooxygenase activity, which inserts molecular oxygen into arachidonic acid to form the intermediate PGG_2, and a peroxidase activity which reduces the hydroperoxide moiety of PGG_2 to the corresponding alcohol and produces PGH_2[2]. This PGH_2 is acted upon by other enzymes to produce the final hormone product, which is secreted from the cell.

The non-steroid anti-inflammatory drugs (NSAIDs) act by inhibiting the COX activity of PGHS[3]. Blocking this activity eliminates the biosynthesis of the prostanoid hormones which mediate the inflammatory response[4]. Since prostanoids are also required for normal physiological functions unrelated to inflammation, the NSAIDs exhibit mechanism-based side effects due to their depression of normal prostanoid levels. It is now clear that prostanoids accompanying the inflammatory burst are produced by a single isoform of COX, COX-2[5]. In contrast, the production of prostanoids associated with housekeeping functions can be ascribed to the activity of the other isoform, COX-1. The discovery of this division of labour has led to the search for inhibitors selective for COX-2[6]. Such inhibitors are expected to lack side effects such as gastric ulceration and internal bleeding which are associated with classical NSAIDs.

COX-1 STRUCTURE

COX-1 can be obtained in large quantities from tissues, whereas COX-2 cannot. Therefore, until recombinant systems became available for the production of COX-2, most biochemical experiments, including structural studies, were carried out with COX-1.

Both COX isoforms are glycoproteins with molecular masses of approximately 70 kDa, and both are haem proteins. COX is an integral membrane protein, COX-1 being located on the luminal side of the endoplasmic reticulum membrane and COX-2 being found in the membranes of the endoplasmic reticulum and nuclear envelope. Both isoforms possess COX and peroxidase activities which are functionally separable, but which may be linked, since oxidizing equivalents generated by the peroxidase reaction may be required to initiate COX turnover. Classical NSAIDs

Figure 1   Ribbon diagrams of COX-1. (a) The COX dimer, viewed perpendicular to the two-fold dimer symmetry axis (vertical in this figure). (b) One of the COX monomers, with the three principal structural domains labelled. The asterisk marks the mouth of the cyclooxygenase channel. The plane of membrane is thought to be horizontal and perpendicular to the plane of the page. The haem may be seen near the top of the molecule (white atoms), as may a flurbiprofen molecule bound in the cyclooxygenase site (black). Part (b) of this figure shows a view of the left monomer of part (a), as seen from the vantage point of the right monomer. Prepared using the program MOLSCRIPT[16]

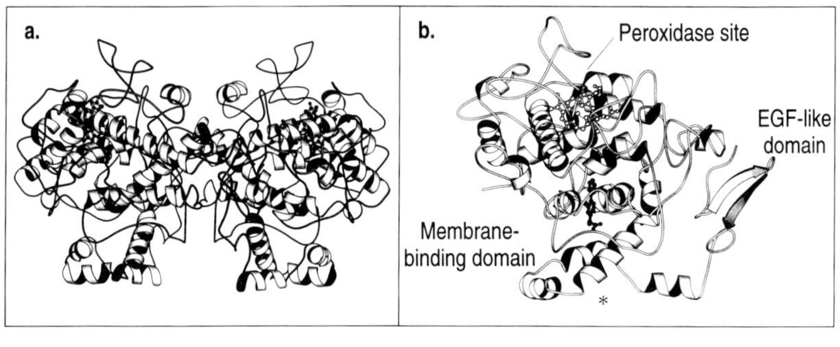

inhibit only the COX activity of both isoforms, leaving the peroxidase activity unaffected.

The X-ray crystal structures of complexes between ovine COX-1 and four different NSAIDs have been determined[7–9]; the current resolution of the best structure is 3.1 Å[10]. These structures show that the enzyme comprises three domains (Figure 1). The first domain is an epidermal growth factor-like (EGF-like) motif found at the N-terminus of the protein. In all structures determined to date, the enzyme forms a symmetrical homodimer, and the EGF-like modules constitute a significant portion of the dimer interface. Thus, the role of this domain is probably to aid in forming a stable dimer, although it is not clear why the enzyme dimerizes. The second structural domain of the protein is the membrane-binding domain, which is made up of four amphipathic helices arrayed along one side of the protein. Unlike their arrangement in soluble proteins, the hydrophobic faces of these helices point outwards, forming a large hydrophobic patch on the surface of the protein. In the dimer, the membrane-binding domains from each monomer are both on the same side of the molecule, and together they form a large surface covered with hydrophobic amino acid side chains which anchors the enzyme to the membrane. The membrane-binding domain probably penetrates only into one leaflet of the bilayer, and does not span the membrane. Hence, COX is a monotopic membrane protein. The third and largest structural domain in COX is the catalytic domain which assumes a canonical haem-dependent peroxidase fold, similar to mammalian myeloperoxidases and, to a lesser extent, to peroxidases from lower eukaryotes[7]. The peroxidase active site is found in

Figure 2   NSAIDs and NSAID analogues for which COX-1 complex structures are known. *(1) flurbiprofen; (2) p-(2'-iodo-5'-thenoyl)-hydrotropic acid; (3) 2-bromoacetoxy-salicylic acid; (4) 1-(4-iodobenzoyl)-5-methoxy-2-methylindole-3-acetic acid*

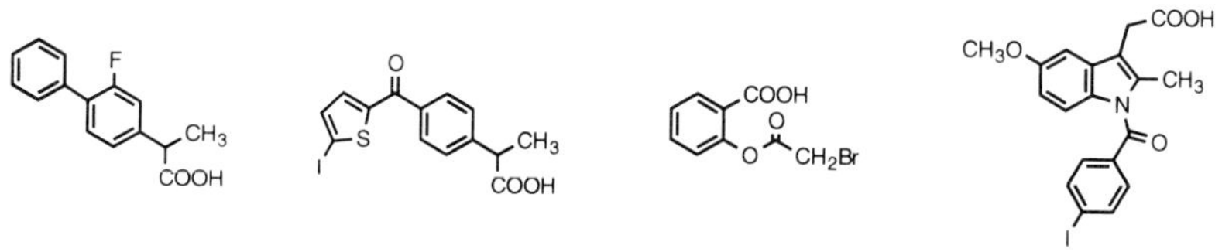

a shallow cleft on the 'top' of the enzyme, i.e. on the side furthest from the membrane. The catalytic domain also contains the COX active site, which is located at the apex of a long, narrow hydrophobic channel which extends upward from the membrane-binding domain into the centre of the catalytic domain. This channel connects the COX active site with the interior of the lipid bilayer, and presumably allows the very hydrophobic substrate arachidonic acid to gain access to the enzyme without passing through a polar environment.

It has long been known that the peroxidase and COX activities of PGHS are functionally separable[11]. This observation is explained by the structure: the two active sites are spatially distinct and unconnected by any channel. Since the PGG_2 produced by the COX reaction is the substrate for the peroxidase reaction, the product must be released by the enzyme and then be bound by the peroxidase site.

THE BINDING OF NSAIDs BY COX-1

Flurbiprofen

The first COX-1 structure determined contained the NSAID flurbiprofen (compound **1** in Figure 2)[7,10]. The aromatic rings of this compound bind in the active site at the apex of the COX channel, directly below Tyr-385, a residue which has been suggested to act as the radical species that abstracts a hydrogen atom from arachidonic acid (see Figure 3). Further down the channel (i.e. closer to the channel mouth), the carboxylate group of the drug forms a salt bridge with Arg-120, one of the only polar residues in the otherwise very hydrophobic COX cavity. Tyr-355 lies close to Arg-120 and also interacts with the carboxylate of the inhibitor. These two residues form a constriction in the channel, burying the flurbiprofen molecule, plugging the channel completely, and preventing the substrate from entering the COX active site. The selectivity of the enzyme for the S-stereoisomer of flurbiprofen can be explained by the structure of the enzyme at this constriction point: the α-methyl group of S-flurbiprofen binds in a small hydrophobic niche lined by leucine and valine residues. The α-methyl group of the R-stereoisomer cannot bind in this small pocket but collides with Tyr-355 instead.

The data for the COX–flurbiprofen complex extend beyond 3.1 Å, and it has been possible to refine the position and orientation of the flurbiprofen molecule with confidence. Not all crystals of COX–NSAID complexes diffract to as high a resolution, however, and in such cases the experimental electron density may not allow the unambiguous determination of the ligand's orientation. To avoid this problem, NSAID analogues labelled with electron-dense heavy atoms were used. The heavy atoms of these analogues can be easily located in even low resolution maps, allowing the orientation of the inhibitor to be assigned with certainty. The three heavy-atom labelled inhibitors used thus far are p-(2'-iodo-5'-thenoyl)-hydrotropic acid (**2**), 2-bromoacetoxy-salicylic acid (**3**), and 1-(4-iodobenzoyl)-5-methoxy-2-methylindole-3-acetic acid (**4**), analogues of suprofen, aspirin and indomethacin, respectively (see Figure 2). All of these compounds are potent COX inhibitors with activities comparable to those of the unlabelled parent compounds.

Iodinated suprofen

Suprofen is a member of the same aryl propionic acid class of NSAIDs to which flurbiprofen belongs, and thus it is not surprising that the modes of binding of iodinated suprofen (**2**) and flurbiprofen (**1**) are very similar[9]. The carboxylic acid group of compound **2** also interacts with Arg-120 and Tyr-355, and the two aromatic rings of the drug project upward from this point, filling the hydrophobic upper section of the COX cavity. The iodine atom on the suprofen analogue packs directly below Tyr-385. Unlike flurbiprofen, suprofen contains a ketone, which should be capable of participating in hydrogen bonds. Indeed, the oxygen atom of this ketone binds close to the side chain of Ser-530, and appears to be hydrogen-bonding to that amino acid's hydroxyl group.

Brominated aspirin

Aspirin is unique among the NSAIDs in that it covalently modifies COX. The structure of COX inactivated by the aspirin analogue **3** illustrates how acetylation of Ser-530 inactivates the enzyme[8], even though this serine does not contribute to catalysis[12]. The bromoacetyl group protrudes outward into the channel, and prevents substrate from diffusing completely up the channel and interacting with Tyr-385. The adduct occupies the same space occupied by flurbiprofen and iodinated suprofen in their respective complexes, suggesting that aspirin and the aryl propionic acids share a common mechanism of blocking substrate access to the catalytic tyrosine through steric hindrance. A surprising result of the determination of the structure of brominated aspirin was the discovery of a salicylic acid molecule bound in the active site channel just below the acetylation site. It was known that the *trans*-esterification reaction by which aspirin acetylates Ser-530 generates salicylic acid as a leaving group; however, because salicylic acid has a much lower affinity for the enzyme than most NSAIDs it was not expected to be observed in the crystal structure. Evidently, the high concentration of drug in the crystallization experiment (~1 mM) allowed the salicylate to bind with high occupancy, since strong electron density was observed for this molecule. The location of the salicylic acid binding site has explained the seemingly paradoxical observation that salicylic acid can antagonize aspirin acetylation of COX at concentrations substantially lower than those at which it inhibits the enzyme. Salicylic acid binds with low affinity to a site in the COX channel, just below Ser-530. Aspirin, because of its structural similarity to salicylic acid, binds to the same site with a comparable affinity, and salicylic acid antagonizes acetylation by competing with aspirin for this site. Even weak binding by aspirin at this site is sufficient to create a high local aspirin concentration in the vicinity of Ser-530, explaining the drug's selectivity for this residue.

Iodinated indomethacin

Indomethacin is one of the most potent NSAIDs, and is widely used in the treatment of rheumatoid arthritis. Because it is such a strong COX inhibitor it is frequently used as a benchmark against which to compare new NSAIDs. Having been used and studied extensively, the compound has achieved the status of a prototypical NSAID, and for this reason the COX–indomethacin complex was considered an important candidate for structural studies. Sustained efforts to crystallize the complex produced many large optically perfect crystals which, however, diffracted X-rays only weakly, suggesting that the COX–indomethacin complex contains some inherent disorder not found in crystals of other complexes.

To examine this possibility, an indomethacin analogue was prepared in which the chlorine atom was replaced by an iodine (iodoindomethacin, **4**). It was possible to introduce this inhibitor into crystals by soaking in buffers containing iodoindomethacin[9]; crystals so prepared diffracted to 4.5 Å. In the resulting difference Fourier maps, the electron-dense iodine atom of the inhibitor was easily located, but the electron density for the remainder of the molecule was weak and discontinuous, and it proved impossible to locate the light atoms of the inhibitor on the basis of the experimental electron density.

The iodine atom of compound **3** binds at the 'top' of the COX active site, at the end of a long narrow channel. Modelling efforts identified two possible conformations for the inhibitor, corresponding to the *cis* and *trans* conformers. Both of these conformations appear equally likely. Conformationally constrained isosteres of indomethacin corresponding to these two conformers are both known to inhibit the enzyme, with only a five-fold difference in potency[15]. It is possible, then, that the COX binding site is plastic, and is capable of binding both the *cis* and *trans* conformations of indomethacin. The binding sites for the two conformers overlap completely, so binding of the two forms is mutually exclusive. If structural rearrangements of the protein associated with the binding of the two conformers differ, then one would expect disorder in crystals of the COX–indomethacin complex, as observed. Structures of complexes of COX with conformationally constrained indomethacin analogues must be determined to address this issue properly.

Figure 3 Close-up view of the cyclooxygenase active site in the COX-1–flurbiprofen complex, seen from the same vantage point as Figure 1b. Part of the haem is seen at top; the peroxidase active site is above the haem, out of the picture. The membrane would be below the bottom of the picture. The drug is shown with white bonds and atoms, outlined in heavy lines. Selected active site residues are also shown. The binding sites for the analogues 2 and 4 and for salicylic acid overlap the flurbiprofen binding site almost completely

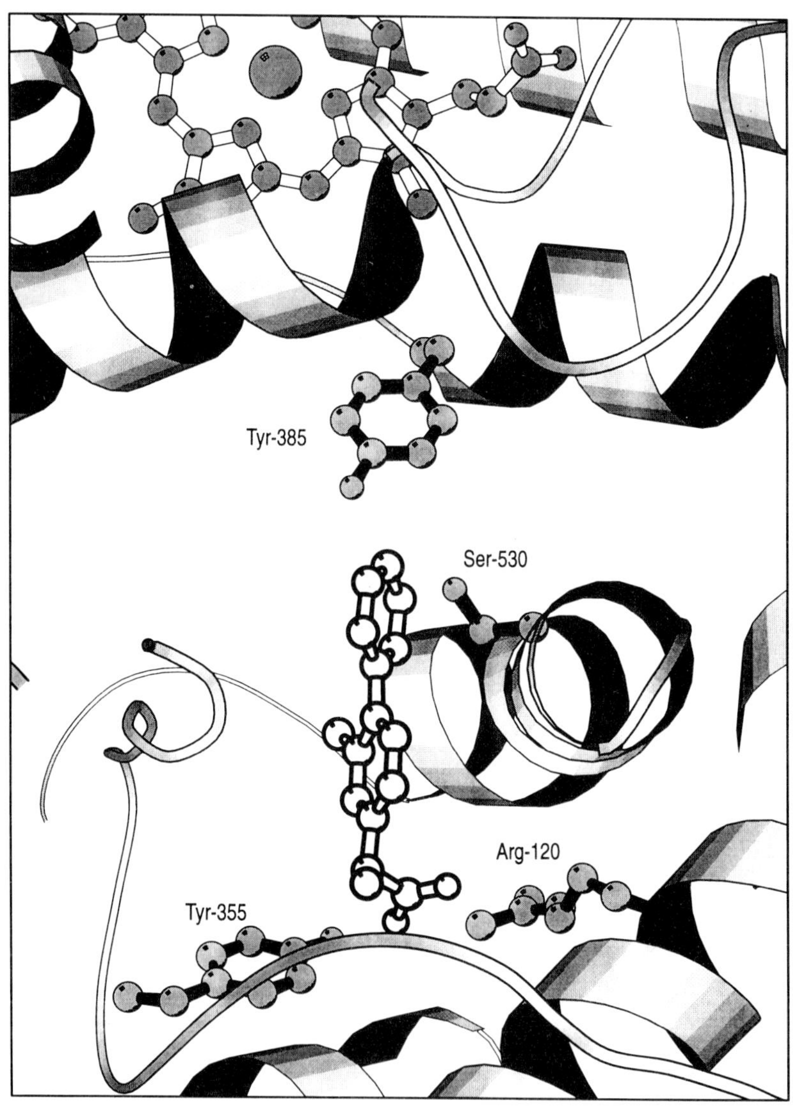

MECHANISTIC IMPLICATIONS OF NSAID BINDING

Arg-120 and Glu-524 are the only charged side chains in the otherwise non-polar COX channel. The fact that Arg-120 forms salt bridges with the carboxylate groups of flurbiprofen, suprofen, salicylic acid and indomethacin suggests that the catalytic role of this side chain may be to position the carboxylate of the arachidonic acid substrate. Model-building studies have demonstrated that placing the carboxylate of arachidonic acid in this fashion enables one to extend the fatty acid chain upward into the COX cavity. When positioned in this way, the fatty acid lies with its carbon-13 atom near Tyr-385. This is consistent with known details of the mechanism, including the fact that the COX reaction is initiated by abstracting the pro-S hydrogen of the fatty acid substrate at carbon-13. Further details of substrate binding, however, may only be forthcoming when the binding of fatty acid to the enzyme has been determined experimentally, since modelling extremely flexible substrates such as arachidonic acid is computationally intractable.

NSAID BINDING AND TIME-DEPENDENT INHIBITION

Many of the NSAIDs, and all of the compounds for which COX-1 complex structures are available, are time-dependent inhibitors; their inhibition is characterized by an apparent increase in inhibitor potency over time[14]. These inhibitors exhibit kinetics consistent with a scheme in which enzyme and inhibitor associate reversibly to form an enzyme–inhibitor complex, which then undergoes an irreversible or pseudo-irreversible conformational change to form a dead-end inactive complex:

$$E + I \rightleftharpoons EI \rightarrow EI^* \text{ or } E + I \rightleftharpoons EI \rightleftharpoons EI^*$$

The precise structural nature of the conformational change accompanying the transition to the EI* complex is not known. The only structures determined to date show either enzyme that has been covalently inactivated by aspirin acetylation or enzyme in complex with inhibitors belonging to the time-dependent class (flurbiprofen, iodosuprofen and iodoindomethacin). We have no picture of the enzyme in an active conformation and therefore no idea of the conformational change(s) exhibited by the enzyme in the course of time-dependent inhibition. In addition, a clear picture of the features which control the mode of inhibition of a given compound has yet to emerge. Very small changes alter the mode of inhibition: for example, the aryl propionic acid flurbiprofen is a time-dependent inhibitor, but its methyl ester is purely competitive. The modes of inhibition of the various NSAIDs are of direct clinical relevance: compounds which are selective for COX-2 are beginning to emerge from drug discovery laboratories, and their selectivity appears to arise from different modes of inhibition toward the two isoforms. Thus, for example, DuP 697 and NS-398 exhibit a roughly 10-fold selectivity for COX-2 over COX-1, and are time-dependent inhibitors of COX-2 but time-independent inhibitors of COX-1[15]. Further work will be required to decipher how this time dependent inhibition occurs and how it might be harnessed for the design of isozyme-specific inhibitors.

IMPLICATIONS FOR THE COX-2 STRUCTURE

The amino acid sequences of COX-1 and COX-2 are only about 60% identical, but the residues lining the active site at the top of the COX channel are almost entirely conserved. Any changes that are found are conservative and unlikely to alter drastically the architecture of the enzyme. It is therefore likely that any differences between the COX sites of the two isoforms are caused by subtle global rearrangements of the protein backbone. The definitive answer must await direct comparison of the COX-1 and COX-2 structures. Until such a time, however, it is intriguing to speculate that differences in the lower section of the COX channel might be important determinants of NSAID selectivity. These regions are more divergent than the COX active site, and, because the channel is so narrow, NSAID binding in this region should block substrate access as effectively as binding in the active site per se.

SUMMARY

The NSAIDs exert their anti-inflammatory, analgesic and antipyretic effects by inhibiting COX. X-ray crystal structures are available for COX-1 in complex with the NSAID flurbiprofen and with heavy-atom labelled analogues of suprofen, aspirin and indomethacin. While structurally diverse, all of these inhibitors bind in the same region of the COX active site, and appear to act by plugging the narrow active site channel and preventing substrate from gaining access.

Acknowledgements

I wish to thank Michael Garavito, in whose laboratory most of this work was accomplished, Daniel Picot, who was the driving force behind the COX-1 structure determination, John Harlan, who assisted tremendously with COX biochemistry, and Opinya Ekabo, who contributed to the synthesis of the NSAID analogues.

References

1. Smith WL, DeWitt DL. Biochemistry of prostaglandin endoperoxide H synthase-1 and synthase-2 and their differential susceptibility to nonsteroidal anti-inflammatory drugs. Semin Nephrol. 1995;15:179–94.
2. Smith WL, Marnett LJ. Prostaglandin endoperoxide synthase: structure and catalysis. Biochim Biophys Acta. 1991;1083:1–17.
3. Mantri P, Witiak DT. Inhibitors of cyclooxygenase and 5-lipoxygenase. Curr Med Chem. 1994; 1:328–55.
4. Vane JR. Inhibition of prostaglandin synthesis as a mechanism of action for aspirin-like drugs. Nature New Biol. 1971;231:232–5.
5. Herschman HR. Regulation of prostaglandin synthase-1 and prostaglandin synthase-2. Cancer Metas Rev. 1994;13:241–56.
6. Vane JR, Botting RM. New insights into the mode of action of anti-inflammatory drugs. Inflamm Res. 1995;44:1–10.
7. Picot D, Loll PJ, Garavito RM. The X-ray crystal structure of the membrane protein prostaglandin H$_2$ synthase-1. Nature. 1994;367:243–9.

8. Loll PJ, Picot D, Garavito RM. The structural basis of aspirin activity inferred from the crystal structure of inactivated prostaglandin H_2 synthase. Nature Struct Biol. 1995;2:637–43.

9. Loll PJ, Picot D, Ekabo O, Garavito RM. The synthesis and use of iodinated non-steroidal antiinflammatory drug analogs as crystallographic probes of the prostaglandin H_2 synthase cyclooxygenase active site. Biochemistry. 1996;35:7330–40.

10. Garavito RM, Picot D, Loll PJ. The 3.1Å X-ray crystal structure of the integral membrane enzyme prostaglandin H_2 synthase-1. Adv Prostaglandin, Thromboxane Leukotriene Res. 1995; 23:99–103.

11. Marshall PJ, Kulmacz RJ. Prostaglandin H synthase: Distinct binding sites for cyclooxygenase and peroxidase substrates. Arch Biochem Biophys. 1988;266:162–70.

12. Shimokawa T, Smith WL. Prostaglandin endoperoxide synthase: The aspirin acetylation region. J Biol Chem. 1992;267:12387–92.

13. Shen TY. Prostaglandin synthetase inhibitors I. In: Vane JR, Ferreira SH, eds. Handbook of Experimental Pharmacology, Vol. 50/II: Anti-Inflammatory Drugs. New York: Springer-Verlag, 1979:316–47.

14. Rome LH, Lands WEM. Structural requirements for time-dependent inhibition of prostaglandin biosynthesis by anti-inflammatory drugs. Proc Natl Acad Sci USA. 1975;72:4863–5.

15. Copeland RA, Williams JM, Biannaras J et al. Mechanism of selective inhibition of the inducible isoform of prostaglandin G/H synthase. Proc Natl Acad Sci USA. 1994;91:11202–6.

16. Kraulis PJ. MOLSCRIPT: A program to produce both detailed and schematic plots of protein structures. J Appl Crystallogr. 1991;24:946–50.

3 Differential inhibition of cyclooxygenases 1 and 2 by NSAIDs

M. PAIRET, L. CHURCHILL and G. ENGELHARDT

The discovery of two isoforms of the cyclooxygenase (COX) enzyme has provided a new impetus for research into anti-inflammatory therapy. Since the demonstration that inhibition of prostanoid synthesis through cyclooxygenase blockade is the mechanism of action of aspirin and related NSAIDs[1], it had been widely accepted that a common mechanism of action can explain both therapeutic and side effects of NSAIDs (Figure 1). The discovery of two isoforms of COX[2-4], a constitutive form (COX-1) and an inducible form (COX-2) led to a refinement of this theory[5,6]. It has recently been proposed that COX-2 is the relevant target for the anti-inflammatory effects of NSAIDs, whereas inhibition of COX-1 is responsible for the gastric and renal side effects as well as for the anti-thrombotic activity of these agents (Figure 2).

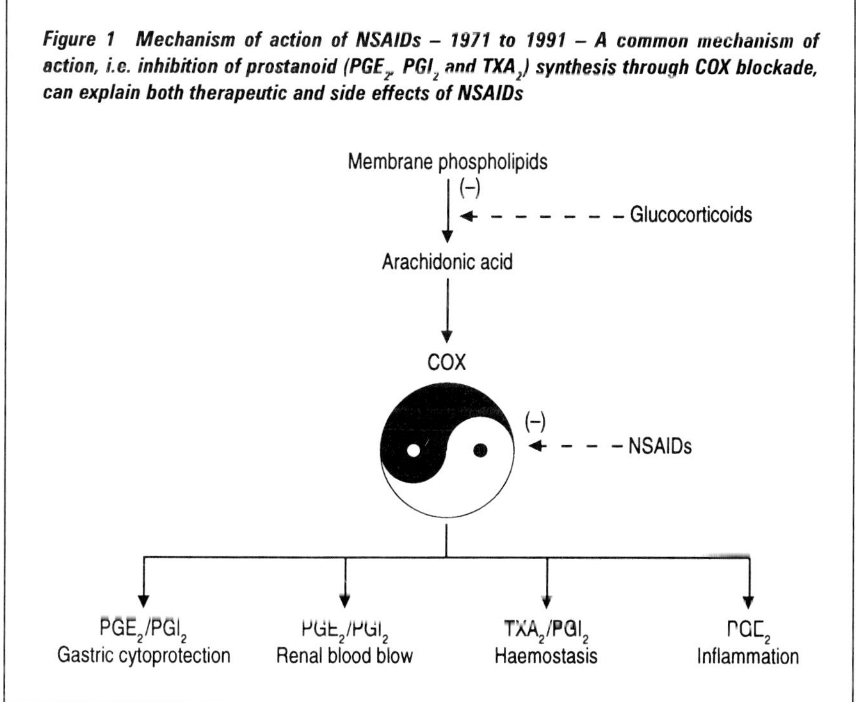

Figure 1 Mechanism of action of NSAIDs – 1971 to 1991 – A common mechanism of action, i.e. inhibition of prostanoid (PGE$_2$, PGI$_2$ and TXA$_2$) synthesis through COX blockade, can explain both therapeutic and side effects of NSAIDs

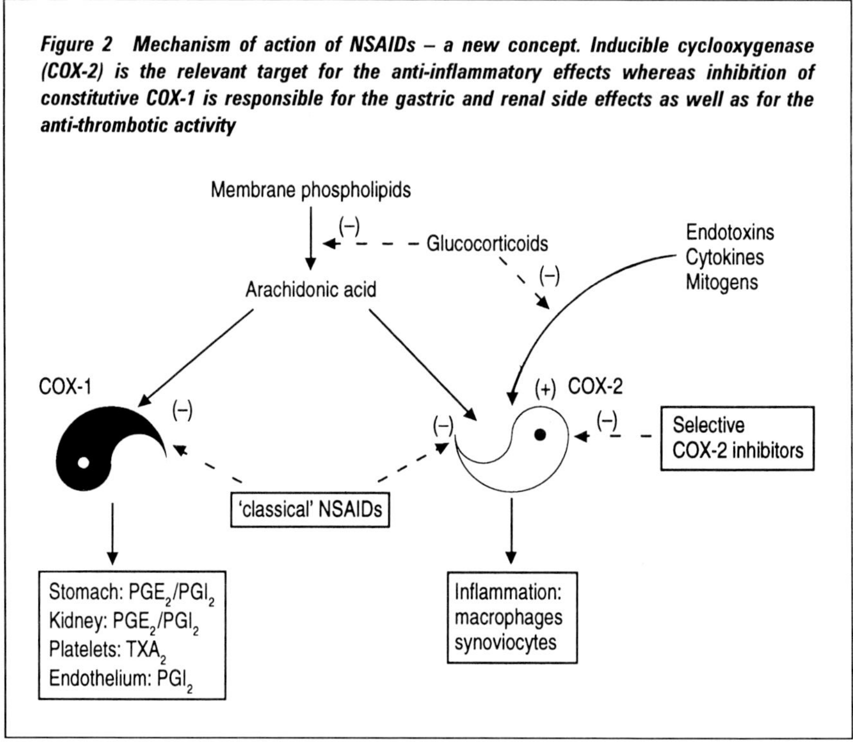

Figure 2   Mechanism of action of NSAIDs – a new concept. Inducible cyclooxygenase (COX-2) is the relevant target for the anti-inflammatory effects whereas inhibition of constitutive COX-1 is responsible for the gastric and renal side effects as well as for the anti-thrombotic activity

This chapter aims to provide an overview of pharmacological results on the relationship between preferential inhibition of COX-2 in vitro and the improved gastric and renal side effect profile in vivo of new NSAIDs. Some important issues such as the value of the experimental models used to test for COX selectivity in vitro, a possible role of COX-1 in inflammation, possible physiological roles of COX-2 and some intriguing results in COX-1/COX-2 knockout mice, will also be analysed.

PREFERENTIAL INHIBITORS OF COX-2

A number of compounds selectively inhibit COX-2 rather than COX-1. Schematically, these compounds can be classified into two groups: those initially selected for development by drug companies because of an improved pharmacological profile in animal models and only later shown to preferentially inhibit COX-2 relative to COX-1, and newly designed COX-2 inhibitors, i.e. substances screened in vitro for their selectivity for COX-2. The latter include SC 58125 (Searle Monsanto)[7] and L-745,337 (Merck Frosst)[8,9]. The former group of compounds includes meloxicam (Boehringer Ingelheim)[10,11], CGP 28238 (Flosulide, Ciba Geigy

Corp)[12,13], NS-398 (Taisho Pharmac Co.)[9,13–17] and DuP 697 (Dupont Co)[13,15]. Selectivity towards COX-2 has also been reported for some compounds in clinical use. An approximately 10-fold selectivity for COX-2 was shown for etodolac in one study investigating time-dependent inhibition using human cells and human recombinant enzymes[18] but no selectivity could be demonstrated in another study when instantaneous inhibition was investigated using human enzymes[19]. Nimesulide also showed selectivity towards COX-2 in three studies using human enzymes or human cells[13,14,20] but not in one study in which murine recombinant enzymes were used[21]. Experimental results in one study using murine recombinant enzymes also suggested that 6-methoxy-2-naphthylacetic acid (6-MNA), the active metabolite of nabumetone, preferentially inhibits COX-2[22]. However, this finding could not be confirmed in other studies in which human enzymes or human cells were used[13,14,19,23].

To illustrate this review we have chosen to present data on meloxicam and flosulide, for which preclinical as well as clinical data are available, on NS-398 and DuP 697, which are widely accepted pharmacological tools and have been used as lead compounds in the structure–activity relationship studies leading to the synthesis of new highly selective COX-2 inhibitors and on L-745,337 and SC 58125, the prototypes of these newly designed selective COX-2 inhibitors.

The differential inhibition of COX-1 and COX-2 by classical NSAIDs and some preferential inhibitors of COX-2 is illustrated in Figure 3. In this model using human recombinant enzymes, standard NSAIDs such as naproxen, preferentially inhibit COX-1, diclofenac is approximately equipotent on both isoforms, meloxicam exhibits a preferential inhibition of COX-2, although some COX-1 inhibitory activity is still present, and SC 58125 is almost completely selective for COX-2.

GASTRIC SPARING EFFECTS OF SELECTIVE COX-2 INHIBITION

Meloxicam

Meloxicam is a typical example covering the evolution of the COX-concept. It was first characterized in vivo in animal models, before the existence of COX-2 was known, and showed potent anti-inflammatory activity in all standard models of inflammation[24]. Comparison of the ulcerogenic dose and the anti-inflammatory dose in a rat model of adjuvant arthritis indicated a superior therapeutic margin in comparison with standard NSAIDs (Table 1)[25]. There was no rationale for this improved pharmacological profile in animals until the discovery of COX-2: preferential inhibition of COX-2 probably explains the higher safety margin of meloxicam over standard NSAIDs. When using unstimulated and LPS stimulated guinea pig macrophages, respectively, as sources of COX-1 and COX-2 activity a selectivity ratio of 0.3 was found. Under the same experimental conditions, diclofenac, indomethacin and piroxicam had selectivity ratios of 2.2, 30 and 34, respectively[10]. Using human recombinant enzymes, IC_{50} values were 2.24 and 0.15 μM for COX-1 and COX-2, respectively, when the enzymes were expressed in cos-cells, and 36.6 and 0.49 μM (ratio IC_{50} COX-2/COX-1: 0.01) in a microsomal assay[11] (Table 2). A 10-fold selectivity for COX-2 over COX-1 has also been demonstrated in a human

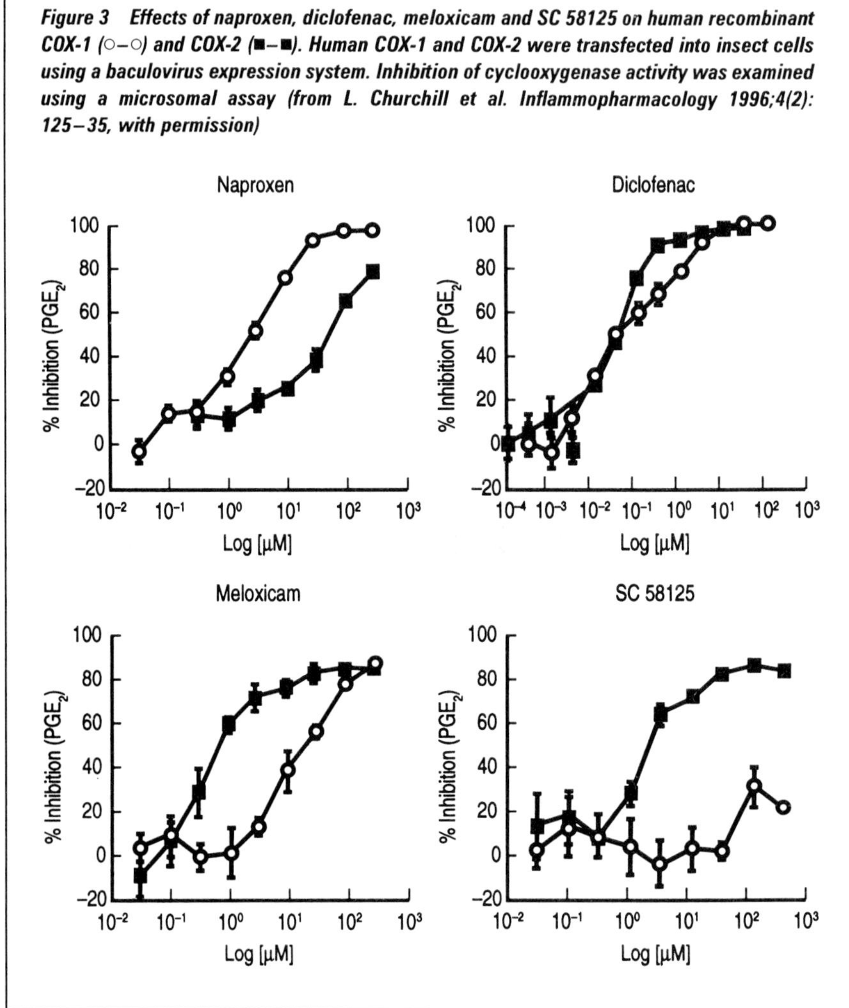

Figure 3 Effects of naproxen, diclofenac, meloxicam and SC 58125 on human recombinant COX-1 (○–○) and COX-2 (■–■). Human COX-1 and COX-2 were transfected into insect cells using a baculovirus expression system. Inhibition of cyclooxygenase activity was examined using a microsomal assay (from L. Churchill et al. Inflammopharmacology 1996;4(2): 125–35, with permission)

whole blood assay[26]. In vivo, in the rat, meloxicam inhibited prostaglandin (PG) biosynthesis more potently at the site of inflammation (carrageenan-induced pleurisy or air pouch) than in the gastric mucosa[27] (Figure 4).

The improved GI tolerability of meloxicam in animals was confirmed in a 4-week double-blind, parallel-group gastroendoscopic study comparing meloxicam 7.5 and 15 mg with placebo and piroxicam 20 mg in human volunteers[28] and by a global safety analysis of data from meloxicam double-blind clinical studies in osteoarthritis (OA) and rheumatoid arthritis (RA), involving more than 3500 patients[29].

Table 1 Comparison of the oral therapeutic indices of NSAIDs in the rat with respect to their ulcerogenic effects on the stomach and their inhibitory effects on the secondary reaction (swelling) in the adjuvant arthritis model (from Engelhardt et al. Inflammation Res. 1995;44:423–33, with permission)

	Dose required to suppress adjuvant arthritis or induce GI erosions				
	Meloxicam	*Diclofenac*	*Naproxen*	*Piroxicam*	*Flurbiprofen*
Adjuvant arthritis $(ID_{50}$ mg/kg$)^a$	0.12	1.24	11.8	0.76	0.97
GI erosions $(ED_{50}$ mg/kg$)^b$	2.47	2.71	11.1	1.07	0.21
Therapeutic index ED_{50}/ID_{50}	20	2.2	0.9	1.4	0.2

Test substances were administered for 3[b] and 21[a] days, respectively.

Table 2 IC_{50} values for the inhibition of recombinant hCOX-1 and hCOX-2 expressed in insect cells using a microsomal assay system (from Churchill et al. Inflammopharmacology 1996;4(2):125–35, with permission)

NSAID	$COX\text{-}1\ IC_{50}$:μM (95% CI)	$COX\text{-}2\ IC_{50}$:μM (95% CI)	Estimated ratio (COX-2/COX-1)
Naproxen	2.7 (1.9–3.4)	~50	18.5
Ibuprofen	13.88 (6.13–21.63)	~80	5.8
Indomethacin	0.10 (0.07–0.13)	0.35 (0.32–0.39)	3.5
6-MNA	~100	NA	–
Diclofenac	0.059 (0.033–0.085)	0.031 (0.022–0.040)	0.5
Nimesulide	~50	9.4 (5.7–13.2)	0.2
Meloxicam	36.6 (26.4–46.8)	0.49 (0.39–0.57)	0.01

NA: <20% inhibition at 300 μM

Flosulide (CGP 28238)

Like meloxicam, the in vivo pharmacology of flosulide was known before COX-2 was characterized. The compound exhibited potent anti-inflammatory activity in adjuvant arthritis (ED_{40}: 0.05 mg/kg p.o.) with improved GI tolerability (threshold dose for GI ulcerogenicity > 30 mg/kg) when compared with standard NSAIDs in the rat[30]. A relative lack of activity against COX-1 was found when using human washed platelets ($IC_{50} > 50\,\mu M$) whereas COX-2 activity from interleukin-1 (IL-1)-stimulated mesangial cells was inhibited with an IC_{50} of 25 nM[12]. Selectivity for COX-2 relative to COX-1 has been confirmed in a human whole blood assay[13].

In a randomized, double-blind, cross-over comparative study in patients suffering from OA, the gastroduodenal tolerability of flosulide 20 mg (t.i.d.) given for 2 weeks, was significantly superior to that of naproxen 500 mg (t.i.d.) for a comparable efficacy[31]. Unfortunately, results of large scale clinical trials are not available since the development of the compound has been discontinued.

Figure 4 *Influence of NSAIDs on PGE_2 content in air pouch exudate (a) and in gastric juice (b) in rats after oral administration. Test substances were administered 25 and 5.5 h before collection of exudate and gastric juice, respectively. Results are expressed as percentage of control value (mean $\pm$ SE). ID_{50} values calculated by regression analysis (95% CI)*

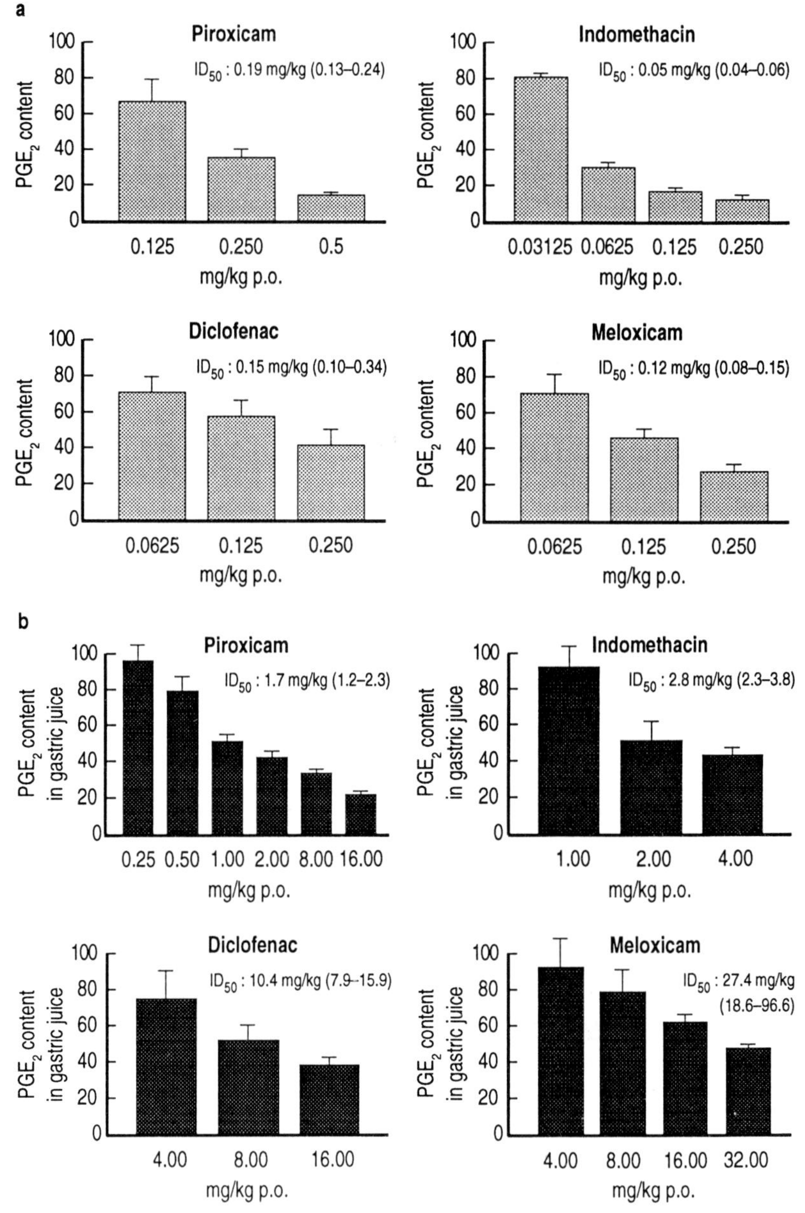

DuP 697

DuP 697 was reported to be a potent inhibitor of paw swelling in adjuvant arthritis with an ID_{50} of 0.2 mg/kg/day p.o. but it did not cause gastric ulcers at doses up to 400 mg/kg p.o. (single administration)[32]. Selective inhibition of COX-2 was later demonstrated using human recombinant enzymes[16] and human cells[13] and is likely to explain the good GI tolerability in the rat.

NS-398

Like DuP 697, NS-398 was first characterized in vivo in the rat where it inhibited PG production in inflamed tissue (carrageenan-air-pouch) more potently (ID_{50}: 0.2 mg/kg p.o.) than in the gastric mucosa (ID_{50}: 62 mg/kg)[33]. In standard models of inflammation, it was almost as potent as indomethacin, and no gastric ulcerations were seen at single oral doses up to 1000 mg/kg[34]. COX-2 selectivity was later demonstrated for the compound in various test systems, including human recombinant enzymes[16] and human cells[9].

L-745,337

L-745,337 is, with SC 58125, a prototype of newly designed selective COX-2 inhibitors. In a human whole cell assay, it was shown to inhibit COX-2 and COX-1 with IC_{50} values of 23 nM and $> 10 \mu M$, respectively[8]. In a human whole blood assay, an IC_{50} ratio for COX-2 relative to COX-1 of < 0.005 was found[9]. In the rat, it inhibited carrageenan-induced oedema with an ED_{30} of 0.2 mg/kg p.o. and prevented hyperalgesia with an ED_{50} of 0.4 mg/kg p.o. without causing gastric ulcerations at doses up to 40 mg/kg. In contrast to indomethacin, no gastrointestinal bleeding was detected in a ^{51}Cr excretion assay in monkeys receiving doses of 10 mg/kg twice daily for 5 days[8].

SC 58125

SC 58125 exhibited a COX-2 selectivity ratio of < 0.005 in studies using mouse[7] or human[35] recombinant enzymes. In the rat, SC 58125 inhibited carrageenan-induced prostaglandin synthesis and paw oedema with ED_{50} values of 0.1 and 10 mg/kg orally, respectively. No inhibition of prostaglandin synthesis by the gastric mucosa and no signs of gastric toxicity were observed at doses up to 10 and 600 mg/kg, respectively[7].

RENAL SPARING EFFECTS OF SELECTIVE COX-2 INHIBITION

In addition to inducing GI erosions, NSAIDs may affect renal function. Most of the unwanted renal effects of NSAIDs, including a reduction of renal blood flow and glomerular filtration rate, water and sodium retention and hyperkalaemia, have been attributed to inhibition of PG synthesis in the kidney[36-38]. Measurement of renal PG synthesis is, therefore, commonly used as a marker of the renal effects of NSAIDs in

Table 3   Influence of NSAIDs on PGE_2 content of pleuritic exudate and urine of rats (from Engelhardt et al. Biochem Pharmacol. 1996;51:29–38, with permission)

| | ID_{50} (mg/kg/day; 95% CI) | | |
NSAID	Pleuritic exudate	Urine	Ratio urine/pleurisy
Meloxicam	0.65 (0.54–0.78)	1.85 (1.05–2.78)	2.8
Diclofenac	5.06 (3.71–6.62)	1.86 (1.23–2.55)	0.37
Piroxicam	0.85 (0.60–1.09)	0.24 (0.10–0.41)	0.28
Flurbiprofen	2.18 (1.78–2.75)	0.26 (0.11–0.58)	0.12
Tenidap	12.8 (9.62–18.0)	0.64 (0.23–1.50)	0.05

preclinical and clinical pharmacology. Table 3 summarizes data comparing the inhibitory activity of some NSAIDs on PG synthesis in the rat, in an inflammatory exudate (carrageenan-induced pleurisy) and in urine. Ratios were calculated by dividing the ID_{50}, i.e. the dose reducing PG synthesis by 50% in the exudate by the dose producing a 50% reduction in urinary PG levels. The rank order of renal sparing activity, indicated by high ratios, parallels the ranking for COX-2 selectivity in vitro[39].

Similarly, NS-398 was much more potent in inhibiting PG synthesis in carrageenan-induced inflammation of the air pouch than in renal papillary tissue in rats, whereas indomethacin was approximately equipotent in both tissues[33]. The renal effects of DuP 697 were also investigated in volume-depleted (furosemide-treated) rats, a model commonly used to mimic the clinical conditions in which cyclo-oxygenase inhibitors, including indomethacin, have been shown to reduce renal blood flow[32]. Unlike indomethacin, DuP 697 did not reduce renal blood flow nor did it potentiate the renal vasoconstrictor effect of angiotensin II. These results support the local production of vasodilatory PG to oppose the effect of renal vasoconstrictors[32]. The renal sparing property of meloxicam was also investigated in healthy female volunteers in a randomized cross-over study with indomethacin as comparator. In contrast to indomethacin (25 mg three times/day) which reduced PGE_2 excretion in urine by approximately 50% (from 47 ± 20 (mean $\pm$ SD) to 24 ± 11 nmol/mol creatinine), meloxicam (7.5 mg/day) showed no significant effect on renal PG synthesis (PGE_2 in urine: 43 ± 28 nmol/mol creatinine)[38].

IMPORTANT ISSUES

The hypothesis that COX-1 is the physiological 'house-keeping' enzyme whereas COX-2 is mainly involved in inflammation is supported by the above pharmacological data. However some critical issues still remain concerning the predictive value of in vitro models used to test for COX-2 selectivity, the role of COX-1 in inflammation and the physiological relevance of COX-2 expression in normal tissue. This point is particularly important in relation to some intriguing new results in knockout mice.

In vitro models to test for COX-2 selectivity

Various experimental models are used to test for COX-1 and COX-2 activity in vitro, including purified enzymes[40], cells transfected with recombinant enzymes[7,16,19,22,41] and intact cell systems[10,12,13,42]. The experimental conditions may vary greatly from one model to the other: various COX-2-inducing agents (lipopolysaccharide, IL-1, etc.) have been used, different incubation times with the test compounds (from a few seconds to 24h) or the COX-2-inducing agent (from 1 to 24h) have been reported, and COX activity has been evaluated by measuring prostaglandin or thromboxane synthesis from either endogenous stores or exogenously administered arachidonic acid. Depending on the model used, absolute IC_{50} values as well as values for the IC_{50} ratio of COX-2 vs COX-1 vary greatly and should not be compared directly. Estimated COX-2/COX-1 ratios range from 0.07 to >75 for indomethacin and from <0.001 to 7.6 for diclofenac. It seems evident from these data that claims for preferential inhibition of COX-2 can only be made when converging comparative data are available from several models.

COX-1 and inflammation

A role of COX-1 in inflammation cannot be excluded: a positive feedback mechanism has been shown between PGE_2 and COX-2[43], COX 1 activity participates in prostaglandin synthesis in both the basal and stimulated states in rat macrophages[44] and an overall increase of COX-1 levels in rheumatoid synovial tissue is likely, due to markedly increased cellularity[45]. We compared the effects on PGE_2 synthesis in an air pouch model in the rat of compounds known to inhibit COX-1 preferentially, such as piroxicam and indomethacin, those known to be equipotent on both isoforms, such as diclofenac, those known to inhibit COX-2 preferentially, such as meloxicam, or those shown to be highly selective for COX-2, such as NS-398 and SC 58125. ID_{50} values were 0.19, 0.05, 0.15, 0.12, 1.48 and 0.80, for piroxicam, indomethacin, diclofenac, meloxicam, NS-398 and SC 58125, respectively. Since the test compounds were administered 25h before exudate collection, the lower efficacy of the selective COX-2 inhibitors NS-398 and SC 58125 may be related to a shorter duration of action in the rat. However, a potent activity is observed for diclofenac, despite the fact that it is known to have a very short half-life in the rat. A role for COX-1 in the induction of COX-2 in the early phase of inflammation may be an alternative explanation. We also studied the degree to which compounds which selectively inhibit COX-2 relative to COX-1, such as meloxicam and SC 58125, can influence symptoms of inflammation and joint destruction in a model of adjuvant arthritis in the rat. Both meloxicam and SC 58125, administered orally once daily for 21 days, dose-dependently inhibited paw swelling. In groups of rats treated with 0.1,

0.3 and 1.0 mg/kg of meloxicam or SC 58125, oedema of the hind paw contralateral to the site of adjuvant administration was reduced to 64, 44 and 29% and to 62, 43 and 31% of the control values, respectively (Figure 5). Systemic signs of inflammation, such as increased erythrocyte sedimentation rate, shift of the serum globulin/albumin ratio, and increase in spleen weight, were also reduced by the two compounds compared with controls, although to a lesser extent than for inflammation of the joint. Radiological and histological assessment of cartilage and bone destruction also revealed a dose-dependent protective effect of the two compounds. Under the experimental conditions used, the degree of protection observed was comparable to that of indomethacin, suggesting a predominant role of COX-2 in the development of immunologically mediated inflammation in rat adjuvant arthritis.

Physiological relevance of COX-2 expression in normal tissue

Although COX-1 predominates in the stomach and kidney, a certain amount of COX-2 has also been observed in the rat[46] and human[47] gastric mucosa as well as in the rat kidney[48]. COX-2 expression in the macula densa is up-regulated in response to restriction of sodium intake in the rat, suggesting that this isoform also plays a regulatory role in the kidney. We therefore investigated the effects of cyclooxygenase inhibition on renin secretion in the rat. Renin secretion was stimulated by pretreatment with furosemide 12 h before the beginning of the experiments (T−12). At T0 the animals received various doses of either indomethacin (0.3, 1, 3 mg/kg p.o.) or SC 58125 (1, 3, 10 mg/kg p.o.) and plasma renin activity (PRA) was measured 4 h later. Both indomethacin and SC 58125 dose-dependently inhibited the furosemide-induced increase in PRA. These results do not parallel the effects of the two compounds on urinary PGE_2: indomethacin reduced urinary PGE_2 with an ID_{50} of approximately 1 mg/kg p.o. whereas much higher doses of SC 58125 were needed (ID_{50}: approx 180 mg/kg p.o.; Figure 6). One explanation for these results may be that urinary PGE_2 reflects COX-1 activity whereas the furosemide-induced increase in PRA reflects COX-2 activity.

A rapid induction of COX activity by luteinizing hormone has also been demonstrated in ovaries[49]. This increased enzymatic activity was shown to be due to inducible COX[50–53], clearly demonstrating a role of this isoform in the induction of ovulation.

The onset of labour in humans is associated with an increase in PG production. Using reverse transcriptase polymerase chain reaction and in situ hybridization techniques, an approximate 100-fold excess of COX-2 relative to COX-1 was demonstrated in human amnion at term[54,55], demonstrating a physiological role for COX-2 in the induction of parturition.

Knockout mice

Mice lacking the COX-1 or COX-2 gene (knockout mice) have recently been produced. As expected, platelets from COX-1 knockout mice are unresponsive to arachidonic-acid-induced aggregation. However, and more surprisingly, these mice

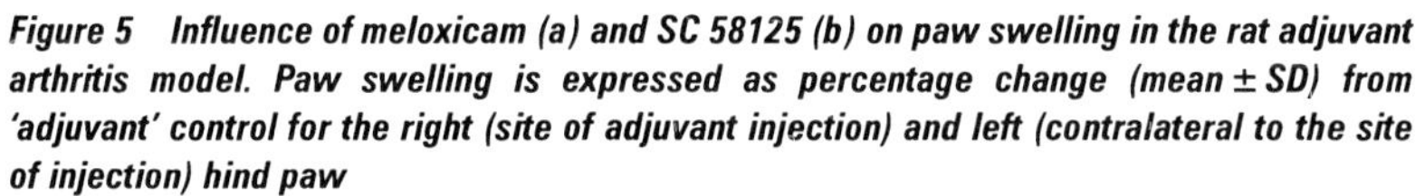

Figure 5   *Influence of meloxicam (a) and SC 58125 (b) on paw swelling in the rat adjuvant arthritis model. Paw swelling is expressed as percentage change (mean ± SD) from 'adjuvant' control for the right (site of adjuvant injection) and left (contralateral to the site of injection) hind paw*

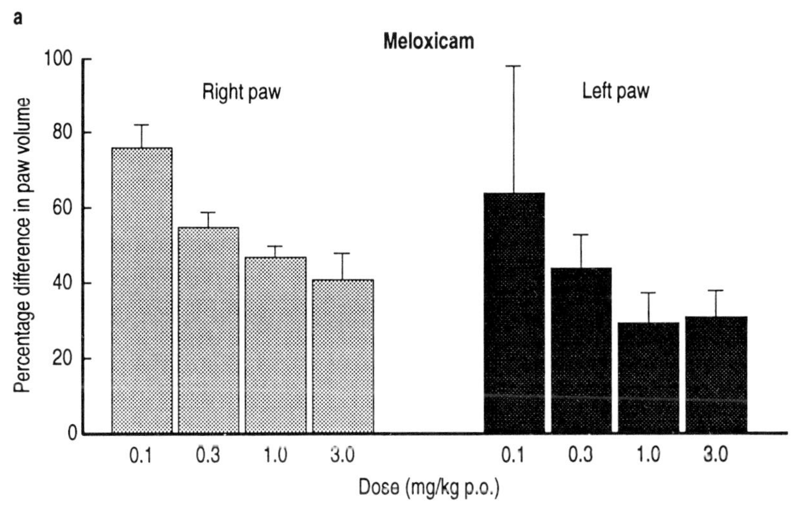

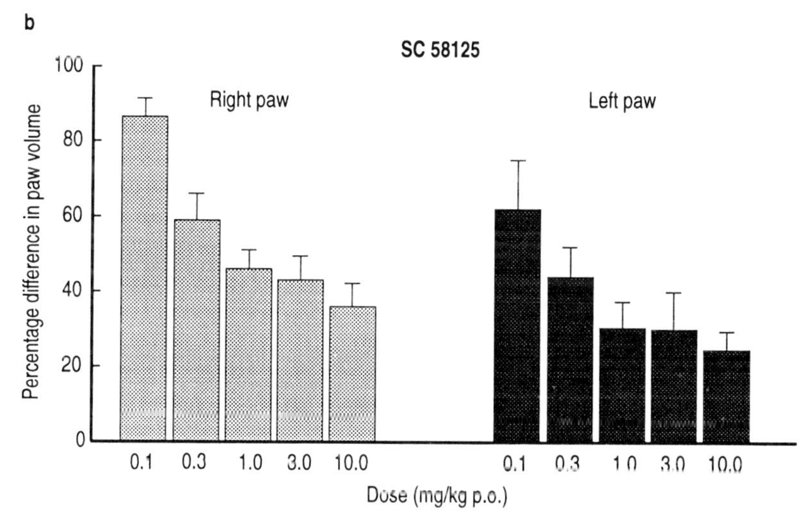

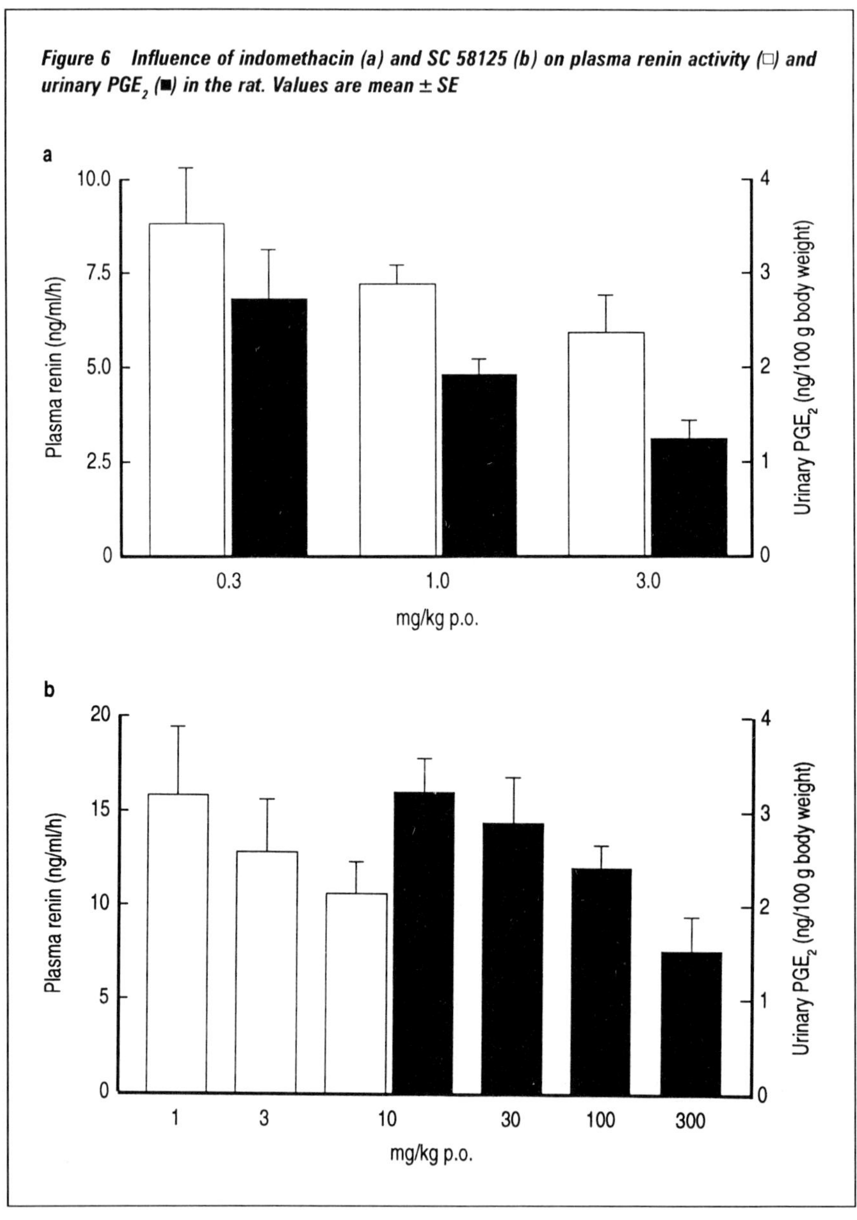

Figure 6   *Influence of indomethacin (a) and SC 58125 (b) on plasma renin activity (□) and urinary PGE$_2$ (■) in the rat. Values are mean ± SE*

did not develop spontaneous stomach ulceration and exhibited an altered acute inflammatory response to arachidonic acid (AA) in the ear swelling assay[56]. Furthermore, COX-2 knockout mice developed a nephropathy and had a normal response in the AA-induced ear swelling assay[57,58]. Although these results do not fit with the theory that COX-1 is the physiological 'house-keeping enzyme' and COX-2 is mainly involved in inflammation, they are not in complete disagreement. The results of the ear inflammation assay can be rationalized since induction of COX-2 is known to occur more than 2 h after inflammatory stimulation. In the experimental conditions used, it is obvious that only COX-1-derived PG can be produced. The nephropathy observed is likely to be the consequence of a lack of maturation of the kidney and will not necessarily occur during treatment with a selective COX-2 inhibitor in animals with a mature kidney. The most unexpected finding is the lack of spontaneous stomach ulceration in COX-1 knockout mice: this might be related to the existence of compensatory mechanisms. It has also been noted that NSAIDs inhibit the COX activity of the prostaglandin H synthase (PGHS) but leave the peroxidase activity unaltered, whereas COX-1 knockout mice are deficient in both of these enzymatic activities[59].

CONCLUSIONS

The good relationship found between selective inhibition of COX-2 relative to COX-1 and improved pharmacological profile in vivo in animals for various NSAIDs supports the hypothesis that selective inhibition of COX-2 may retain the anti-inflammatory activity while minimizing gastric and renal side effects. Large scale clinical results are only available for meloxicam: they show clearly a reduced GI toxicity in comparison to standard NSAIDs which has now to be confirmed in post-marketing surveillance studies. A careful analysis of efficacy/safety data in both osteoarthritis and rheumatoid arthritis for compounds in clinical use for which a preferential inhibition of COX-2 has been suggested, such as nimesulide and etodolac, is needed. Furthermore, since the aforementioned agents still retain some COX-1 inhibitory activity, clinical data on specific COX-2 inhibitors such as L-745,337 and SC 58125 are necessary to test the hypothesis that COX-2 inhibition is the only relevant target of the anti-inflammatory activity of NSAIDs whereas COX-1 inhibition is responsible for their gastric and renal side effects.

Additional experimental studies are also needed to investigate a possible role of COX-1 in inflammation and the physiological relevance of COX-2 expression in normal tissues. Such investigations may help to predict not only potential adverse effects but also new therapeutic indications for selective COX-2 inhibitors. Indeed, experimental results already suggest a role for COX-2 in various pathological conditions, such as pain[60,61], neuronal injury[62,63], asthma[64], preterm delivery[65,66] and large bowel adenomas and/or carcinomas[67-69].

References

1. Vane JR. Inhibition of prostaglandin synthesis as a mechanism of action of aspirin-like drugs. Nature New Biol. 1971;231:232–5.
2. Fu JY, Masferrer JL, Seibert K, Raz A, Needleman P. The induction and suppression of prostaglandin H₂ synthase (cyclooxygenase) in human monocytes. J Biol Chem. 1990;265:16737–40.

3. Xie W, Chipman JG, Robertson DL, Erikson RL, Simmons DL. Expression of a mitogen-responsive gene encoding prostaglandin synthase is regulated by mRNA splicing. Proc Natl Acad Sci USA. 1991;88:1692–6.
4. Hla T, Neilson K. Human cyclooxygenase-2 cDNA. Proc Natl Acad Sci USA. 1992;89:7384–8.
5. Vane JR. Towards a better aspirin. Nature. 1994;367:215–16.
6. Pairet M, Engelhardt G. Distinct isoforms (COX-1 and COX-2) of cyclooxygenase: possible physiological and therapeutic implications. Fund Clin Pharmacol. 1996;10:1–15.
7. Seibert K, Zhang Y, Leahy K et al. Pharmacological and biochemical demonstration of the role of cyclooxygenase 2 in inflammation and pain. Proc Natl Acad Sci USA. 1994;91: 12013–17.
8. Chan CC, Boyce R, Brideau C et al. Pharmacology of a selective cyclooxygenase-2 inhibitor, I-745,337: A novel nonsteroidal anti-inflammatory agent with an ulcerogenic sparing effect in rat and nonhuman primate stomach. J Pharmacol Exp Ther. 1995;274:1531–7.
9. Panara MR, Greco A, Santini G et al. Effects of the novel anti-inflammatory compounds, N-[-(cyclohexyloxy)-4-nitrophenyl]methanesulfonamide (NS-398) and 5-methanesulfonamido-6(2,4-difluorothiophenyl)-1-indanone (L-745,337), on the cyclooxygenase activity of human blood prostaglandin endoperoxide synthases. Br J Pharmacol. 1995;116:2429–34.
10. Engelhardt G, Bögel R, Schnitzler C, Utzmann R. Meloxicam: influence on arachidonic acid metabolism: Part 1. In vitro findings. Biochem Pharmacol. 1996;51:21–8.
11. Churchill L, Graham A, Shih CK, Pauletti D, Farina PR, Grob P. Selective inhibition of human cyclooxygenase-2 by meloxicam. Inflammopharmacology. 1996;4:125–35.
12. Klein T, Nüsing RM, Pfeilschifter J, Ullrich V. Selective inhibition of cyclooxygenase 2. Biochem Pharmacol. 1994;48:1605–10.
13. Grossman CJ, Wiseman J, Lucas FS, Trevethick MA, Birch PJ. Inhibition of constitutive and inducible cyclooxygenase activity in human platelets and mononuclear cells by NSAIDs and COX 2 inhibitors. Inflamm Res. 1995;44:253–7.
14. Barnett J, Chow J, Ives D et al. Purification, characterization and selective inhibition of human prostaglandin G/H synthase 1 and 2 expressed in the baculovirus system. Biochim Biophys Acta. 1994;1209:130–9.
15. Futaki N, Takahashi S, Yokoyama M, Arai I, Higuchi S, Otomo S. NS-398, a new anti-inflammatory agent, selectively inhibits prostaglandin G/H synthase/cyclooxygenase (COX-2) activity in vitro. Prostaglandins. 1994;47:55–9.
16. Gierse JK, Hauser SD, Creely DP et al. Expression and selective inhibition of the constitutive and inducible forms of human cyclo-oxygenase. Biochem J. 1995;305:479–84.
17. Oullet M, Percival MD. Effect of inhibitor time-dependency and selectivity towards cyclo-oxygenase isoforms. Biochem J. 1995;306:247–51.
18. Glaser K, Sung ML, O'Neill K et al. Etodolac selectively inhibits human prostaglandin G/H synthase-2 (PGHS-2) versus human PGHS-1. Eur J Pharmacol. 1995;281:107–11.
19. Laneuville O, Breuer DK, Dewitt DL, Hla T, Funk CD, Smith WD. Differential inhibition of human prostaglandin endoperoxide H synthases-1 and -2 by nonsteroidal anti-inflammatory drugs. J Pharmacol Exp Ther. 1994;271:927–34.
20. Tavares IA, Bishai PM, Bennett A. Activity of nimesulide on constitutive and inducible cyclooxygenases. Arzneim Forsch. 1995;45:1093–5.
21. Huff R, Collins P, Kramer S et al. A structural feature of N-[2-(cyclohexyloxy)-4-nitrophenyl]methanesulfonamide (NS-398) that governs its selectivity and affinity for cyclooxygenase 2 (COX2). Inflamm Res. 1995;Suppl 2:S145–6.
22. Meade EA, Smith WL, DeWitt DL. Differential inhibition of prostaglandin endoperoxide synthase (cyclooxygenase) isozymes by aspirin and other non-steroidal anti-inflammatory drugs. J Biol Chem. 1993;268:6610–14.
23. Patrignani P, Panara MR, Greco A et al. Biochemical and pharmacological characterization of the cyclooxygenase activity of human blood prostaglandin endoperoxide synthases. J Pharmacol Exp Ther. 1994;271:1705–10.
24. Engelhardt G, Homma D, Schlegel K, Utzmann R, Schnitzler C. Anti-inflammatory, analgesic, antipyretic and related properties of meloxicam, a new non-steroidal anti-inflammatory agent with favourable gastrointestinal tolerance. Inflamm Res. 1995;44:423–33.
25. Engelhardt G, Homma D, Schnitzler C. Meloxicam: a potent inhibitor of adjuvant arthritis in the Lewis rat. Inflamm Res. 1995;44:548–55.

26. Pairet M, Engelhardt G. Differential inhibition of COX-1 and COX-2 in vitro and pharmacological profile in vivo of NSAIDs. In: J Vane, J Botting, R Botting, editors. Improved Non-steroidal Anti-inflammatory Drugs – COX-2 Enzyme Inhibitors. Dordrecht: Kluwer Academic, 1996:103–19.

27. Engelhardt G, Bögel R, Schnitzler C, Utzmann R. Meloxicam: influence on arachidonic acid metabolism. Part 2. In vivo findings. Biochem Pharmacol. 1996;51:29–38.

28. Patoia L, Santucci L, Furno P et al. A 4-week, double-blind, parallel-group study to compare the gastrointestinal effects of meloxicam 7.5 mg, meloxicam 15 mg, piroxicam 20 mg and placebo by means of faecal blood loss, endoscopy and symptom evaluation in healthy volunteers. Br J Rheumatol. 1996;35(Suppl 6):61–7.

29. Distel M, Mueller C, Bluhmki E, Fries J. Safety of meloxicam, a global analysis of clinical trials. Br J Rheumatol. 1996;35(Suppl 6):68–77.

30. Wiesenberg-Boettcher I, Schweizer A, Green JR, Mueller K, Maerki F, Pfeilschifter J. The pharmacological profile of CGP 28238, a novel highly potent anti-inflammatory compound. Drugs Exp Clin Res. 1989;15:501–9.

31. Bjarnason I, Hayllar J, Parker J, Schupp J, Macpherson A. A randomised, double blind, crossover comparative endoscopy study on gastroduodenal tolerability of flosulide and naproxen. Gastroenterology. 1994;106(Suppl 4):A53.

32. Gans KR, Gabraight W, Roman RJ et al. Anti-inflammatory and safety profile of DuP 697, a novel orally effective prostaglandin synthesis inhibitor. J Pharmacol Exp Ther. 1990;254: 180–7.

33. Futaki N, Arai I, Hamasaka Y, Takahashi S, Higuchi S, Otomo S. Selective inhibition of NS-398 on prostanoid production in inflamed tissue in rat carrageenan–air-pouch inflammation. J Pharm Pharmacol. 1992;45:735–55.

34. Futaki N, Yoshikawa K, Hamasaka Y et al. NS-398, a novel non-steroidal anti-inflammatory drug with potent analgesic and antipyretic effects, which causes minimal stomach lesions. Gen Pharmacol. 1993;24:105–10.

35. Reitz DB, Li JL, Norton MB et al. Selective cyclooxygenase inhibitors: novel 1,2-diarylcyclopentenes are potent and orally active COX-2 inhibitors. J Med Chem. 1994;37:3878–81.

36. Carmichael J, Shankel SW. Effects of nonsteroidal anti-inflammatory drugs on prostaglandins and renal function. Am J Med. 1985;78:992–1000.

37. Murray MD, Brater DC. Renal toxicity of nonsteroidal anti-inflammatory drugs. Annu Rev Pharmacol Toxicol. 1993;32:435–65.

38. Frölich JC, Stichtenoth DO. Renal side effects of NSAID: can they be avoided? In: J Vane, J. Botting, R. Botting, editors. Improved Non-steroidal Anti-inflammatory Drugs – COX-2 Enzyme Inhibitors. Dordrecht: Kluwer Academic, 1996:203–28.

39. Engelhardt G. Pharmacology of meloxicam, a new non-steroidal anti-inflammatory drug with an improved safety profile through preferential inhibition of COX-2. Br J Rheumatol. 1996;35 (Suppl 6):in press.

40. Futaki N, Takahashi S, Yokoyama M, Arai I, Higuchi S, Otomo S. NS-398, a new anti-inflammatory agent, selectively inhibits prostaglandin G/H synthase/cyclooxygenase (COX-2) activity in vitro. Prostaglandins. 1994;47:55–9.

41. O'Neill GP, Mancini JA, Kargman S et al. Overexpression of human prostaglandin G/H synthase-1 and -2 by recombinant vaccinia virus: inhibition by nonsteroidal anti-inflammatory drugs and biosynthesis of 15-hydroxyeicosatetraenoic acid. Mol Pharmacol. 1994;45:245–54.

42. Mitchell JA, Akarasereenont P, Thiemermann C, Flower RJ, Vane JR. Selectivity of nonsteroidal antiinflammatory drugs as inhibitors of constitutive and inducible cyclooxygenase. Proc Natl Acad Sci USA. 1994;90:11693–7.

43. Mertz PM, DeWitt DL, Stetler-Stevenson WG, Wahl LM. Interleukin 10 suppression of monocyte prostaglandin H synthase-2. J Biol Chem. 1994;269:21322–9.

44. Wilborn J, DeWitt DL, Peters-Golden M. Expression and role of cyclooxygenase isoforms in alveolar and peritoneal macrophages. Am J Physiol. 1995;268:L294–301.

45. Crofford L. Expression and regulation of COX-2 synovial tissues of arthritic patients. In: J Vane, J. Botting, R. Botting, editors. Improved Non-steroidal Anti-inflammatory Drugs – COX-2 Enzyme Inhibitors. Dordrecht: Kluwer Academic, 1996:133–44.

46. Iseki S. Immunocytochemical localization of cyclooxygenase-1 and cyclooxygenase 2 in the rat stomach. Histochem J. 1995;27:323–8.

47. O'Neill GP, Ford-Hutchinson AW. Expression of mRNA for cyclooxygenase-1 and cyclo-oxygenase-2 in human tissues. FEBS Lett. 1993;330:156–60.
48. Harris RC, McKanna JA, Akai Y, Jacobson HR, Dubois RN, Breyer MD. Cyclooxygenase-2 is associated with the macula densa of rat kidney and increases with salt restriction. J Clin Invest. 1994;94:2504–10.
49. Wong WYL, DeWitt DL, Smith WL, Richards JS. Rapid induction of prostaglandin endoperoxide synthase induced by luteinizing hormone and cAMP is blocked by inhibitors of transcription and translation. Mol Endocrinol. 1989;3:1714–23.
50. Wong WYL, Richards JS. Evidence for two antigenically distinct molecular weight variants of prostaglandin H synthase in the rat ovary. Mol Endocrinol. 1991;5:1269–79.
51. Sirois J, Simmons DL, Richards JS. Hormonal regulation of messenger ribonucleic acid encoding a novel isoform of prostaglandin endoperoxide H synthase in rat preovulatory follicles. J Biol Chem. 1992;267:11586–92.
52. Sirois J, Richards JS. Transcriptional regulation of the rat prostaglandin endoperoxide synthase 2 gene in granulosa cells. J Biol Chem. 1993;268:21931–8.
53. Sirois J, Levy LO, Simmons DL, Richards JS. Characterization and hormonal regulation of the promoter of the rat prostaglandin endoperoxide synthase 2 gene in granulosa cells. J Biol Chem. 1993;268:7384–5.
54. Slater D, Berger L, Newton R, Moore G, Bennett P. The relative abundance of type 1 to type 2 cyclo-oxygenase mRNA in human amnion at term. Biochem Biophys Res Commun. 1994; 198:304–8.
55. Slater D, Berger L, Newton R, Moore G, Bennett P. Expression of cyclooxygenase types 1 and 2 in human fetal membranes at term. Am J Obstet Gynecol. 1995;172:77–82.
56. Langenbach R, Morham SG, Tiano HF et al. Prostaglandin synthase 1 gene disruption in mice reduces arachidonic acid-induced inflammation and indomethacin-induced gastric ulceration. Cell. 1995;83:483–92.
57. Morham SG, Langenbach R, Loftin CD et al. Prostaglandin synthase 2 gene disruption causes severe renal pathology in the mouse. Cell. 1995;83:473–82.
58. Dinchuk JE, Car BD, Focht RJ et al. Renal abnormalities and an altered inflammatory response in mice lacking cyclooxygenase II. Nature. 1995;378:406–9.
59. DeWitt D, Smith WL. Yes, but do they still get headaches? Cell. 1995;83:345–8.
60. Yamagata K, Andreasson KI, Kaufmann WE, Barnes CA, Worley PF. Expression of a mitogen-inducible cyclooxygenase in brain neurons: regulation by synaptic activity and glucocorticoids. Neuron. 1993;11:371–86.
61. Breder CD, DeWitt D, Kraig RP. Characterization of inducible cyclooxygenase in rat brain. J Comp Neurol. 1995;355:296–315.
62. Bazan NG, Fletcher BS, Herschman HR, Mukherjee PK. Platelet-activating factor and retinoic acid synergistically activate the inducible prostaglandin synthase gene. Proc Natl Acad Sci USA. 1994;91:5252–6.
63. Chen Y, Marsh T, Zhang JS, Graham SH. Expression of cyclooxygenase 2 in rat brain following kainate treatment. NeuroReport. 1995;6:245–8.
64. Mitchell JA, Belvisi MG, Akarasereenont PA et al. Induction of cyclo-oxygenase-2 by cytokines in human pulmonary epithelial cells: regulation by dexamethasone. Br J Pharmacol. 1994;113: 1008–14.
65. Ishihara O, Matsuoka K, Kinoshita K, Sullivan MHF, Elder MG. Interleukin-1β-stimulated PGE_2 production from early first trimester human decidual cells is inhibited by dexamethasone and progesterone. Prostaglandins. 1995;49:15–26.
66. Silver RM, Edwin SS, Trautman MS et al. Bacterial lipopolysaccharide-mediated fetal death: production of a newly recognized form of inducible cyclooxygenase (COX-2) in murine decidua in response to lipopolysaccharide. J Clin Invest. 1995;95:725–31.
67. Eberhardt CE, Coffey RJ, Radhika A, Giardiello FM, Ferrenbach S, Dubois R. Up-regulation of cyclooxygenase 2 gene expression in human colorectal adenomas and carcinomas. Gastroenterology. 1994;107:1183–8.
68. Kargman SL, O'Neill GP, Vickers PJ, Evans JF, Mancini JA, Jothy S. Expression of prostaglandin G/H synthase-1 and -2 protein in human colon cancer. Cancer Res. 1995;55:2556–9.
69. Tsuji M, DuBois RN. Alterations in cellular adhesion and apoptosis in epithelial cells overexpressing prostaglandin endoperoxide synthase 2. Cell. 1995;83:493–501.

4 Blockade of inflammatory hyperalgesia and cyclooxygenase-2

S. H. FERREIRA

Although the final peripheral hyperalgesic mediators in most inflammatory reactions are cyclooxygenase (COX) products a cascade of cytokines precedes their release. At the onset of the inflammatory response resident cells, particularly macrophages, act as alarm cells, signalling the presence of foreign or deleterious stimuli via the release of cytokines. Using specific antisera and COX inhibitors we have demonstrated that interleukin-1β (IL-1β) is a key cytokine for the release of prostaglandins (PG). The release of IL-1β is preceded by the liberation of other cytokines such as tumour necrosis factor-α (TNFα) and interleukin-6 (IL-6). In inflammation increased production of PG is thought to result from the induction of phospholipase A_2 (PLA_2) and/or COX-2 by IL-1β. However, local administration into the paw of arachidonic acid in a dose that does not itself cause hyperalgesia strongly potentiates the intraplantar effect of IL-1β or carrageenan, suggesting that induction of COX-2 is a limiting process in the development of inflammatory hyperalgesia. Induction of COX-2 is typically inhibited by corticosteroids. In our system IL-1β-induced hyperalgesia is inhibited by dexamethasone through the release of lipocortin.

The importance of COX-2 for inflammatory pain is supported by the fact that selective COX-2 inhibitors have potent antinociceptive effects. In the present study we found that meloxicam, a selective COX-2 inhibitor, does not affect PG-induced hyperalgesia but has a strong inhibitory effect on the arachidonic acid induced potentiation of rat paw hyperalgesia induced by IL-1β or carrageenan.

CYCLOOXYGENASE

Despite the many analgesics available to the modern clinician it is often difficult to find the ideal analgesic for a specific patient. Although they are highly effective, centrally acting analgesics have behavioural side effects, and the use of non-steroid anti-inflammatory COX inhibitors (NSAIDs) is often limited by their inherent and undesirable nephrotoxic and gastrointestinal effects. During the last three decades the basic physiopathological and molecular mechanisms involved in central and peripheral pain have begun to be unravelled. It is hoped that this knowledge will reveal new targets for the development of better analgesic drugs.

Two isoforms of COX have been identified[1]. COX-1 is a constitutive enzyme producing PG that are protective in the gastrointestinal tract and kidney, whereas the inducible enzyme COX-2 produces PG that participate in the inflammatory response. COX-2 is induced by a variety of pro-inflammatory stimuli, particularly cytokines. Because of the association of COX-1 inhibition with gastric problems, selective

COX-2 inhibitors became a target for development of a new anti-inflammatory drug with a profile different from that of the majority of classical NSAIDs which inhibit both isoforms[2]. This approach is apparently in contradiction with the observation that disruption of the gene encoding COX-1 in the mouse was followed by a decreased inflammatory response to arachidonic acid[3]. Conversely, disruption of COX-2 gene had no effect on inflammatory responses[4,5]. Nevertheless, selective COX-2 inhibitors show potent antinociceptive effects[6,7].

PROSTAGLANDIN HYPERALGESIA

Our early hypothesis that aspirin-like drugs (NSAID), prevent receptor sensitization because they inhibit PG[8] is now widely accepted. The ability of PGE_2 and PGI_2 to sensitize pain receptors has been extensively studied and demonstrated in man and in animals, using both behavioural and electrophysiological techniques[9]. Sensitization of the pain receptor is common to all types of inflammatory pain. C-polymodal, high threshold receptors, or receptors connected by fine myelinated fibres, have long been associated with inflammatory hyperalgesia. Over recent years, a new 'sleeping' nociceptor associated with a small afferent fibre has been described in deep visceral innervation (colon and bladder) and in joints[10]. Sleeping nociceptors cannot be activated in normal tissues but are switched on during inflammation. The functional up-regulation of the pain receptors, clinically referred to as hyperalgesia, causes previously ineffective stimuli to become painful.

BIOCHEMICAL EVENTS AND HYPERALGESIA

The molecular events associated with hyperalgesia are not yet fully understood. However, there is evidence that an increase in $cAMP/Ca^{2+}$ concentrations is associated with the functional up-regulation of nociceptors. We have shown that administration of dibutyryl cAMP, Ca^{2+} ionophore or $BaCl_2$ (which increases the concentration of free Ca^{2+} in the cytosol) into the rat paw causes hyperalgesia. Administration of PG or sympathomimetics (noradrenaline or dopamine), agents known to stimulate neuronal cAMP synthesis, also causes hyperalgesia. On the other hand, pretreatment of the paws with a calcium channel blocker or with lanthanum (which blocks Ca^{2+} influx) prevents the development of this hyperalgesia[11]. The hypothesis that hyperalgesia occurs subsequent to an increase in cytosolic $cAMP/Ca^{2+}$ concentrations has received the experimental support of other groups using different hyperalgesic tests[12,13]. The final biochemical events responsible for the functional up-regulation of the nociceptor are not yet understood. The mechanism may involve the activation of a protein kinase A[13], with subsequent phosphorylation of an ion channel, or the modulation of cytosolic structures that control intracellular calcium levels. Molecular events occurring in the primary sensory neurones seem to be maintained via retrograde stimulation by a continuous release of glutamate in the spinal cord during inflammatory hyperalgesic processes[14].

There is, however, a biochemical system which is able to down-regulate sensitized nociceptors. Direct blockade of ongoing hyperalgesia was observed after local administration of dibutyryl cGMP, or by substances which stimulate neuronal guanylate cyclase (carbachol or nitric oxide generators)[15–18]. Thus it seems that the functional up- or down-regulation of the nociceptors is dependent on a balance between nociceptor cAMP/cGMP content. Some peripheral acting analgesics such as dipyrone, diclofenac or peripheral opiates have been described as acting in this way via stimulation of the arginine/nitric oxide system present in the primary sensory neurone[18].

CYTOKINES AND BRADYKININ IN THE RELEASE OF HYPERALGESIC AGONISTS

Although PG are among the final peripheral hyperalgesic mediators in most types of inflammation, many other mediators precede PG release. At the onset of the inflammatory response, the macrophage may act as the initial trigger, signalling the presence of noxious stimuli via the release of cytokines[19–22]. This cytokine release seems to constitute the link between cellular injury and/or recognition of non-self and the liberation of the 'direct acting' mediators responsible for the development of local and systemic inflammatory signs and symptoms. Using specific antisera for IL-1β and IL-8, cyclooxygenase inhibitors and sympatholytic drugs, we have demonstrated that these cytokines are responsible for the prostaglandin and sympathomimetic components in experimental animal models. In inflammation, TNFα release precedes, and probably initiates, the release of IL-1β and IL-8[22].

Work from various laboratories, including ours, shows that bradykinin, rather than acting as a receptor activator, may contribute to inflammatory hyperalgesia by releasing PG and sympathomimetic amines via the release of hyperalgesic cytokines. We found that bradykinin-induced hyperalgesia is mediated by TNFα, which in turn stimulates the release of the hyperalgesic cytokines IL-8 and IL-1. Hyperalgesia induced by carrageenan and LPS is similarly mediated by the release of bradykinin and TNFα. In the presence of a high concentration of LPS, the importance of bradykinin is overshadowed by the direct release of cytokines[23].

It is now well established that during inflammation the induction of PG production is the result of the release of cytokines and growth factors, and that these substances are able to induce the activity of COX-2.

OBJECTIVE

Data are presented here supporting the suggestion that the COX associated with inflammatory hyperalgesia is inducible and shares some of the characteristics of COX-2. The importance of COX-2 in inflammation is supported by the fact that several COX-2 preferential inhibitors are not only potent antinociceptives but also prevent development of oedema in the rat paw[2,6,24]. Meloxican, a preferential COX-2 inhibitor, reduces dose-dependently the hyperalgesia induced by IL-1β and carrageenan, and also inhibits carrageenan-induced oedema (Figure 1).

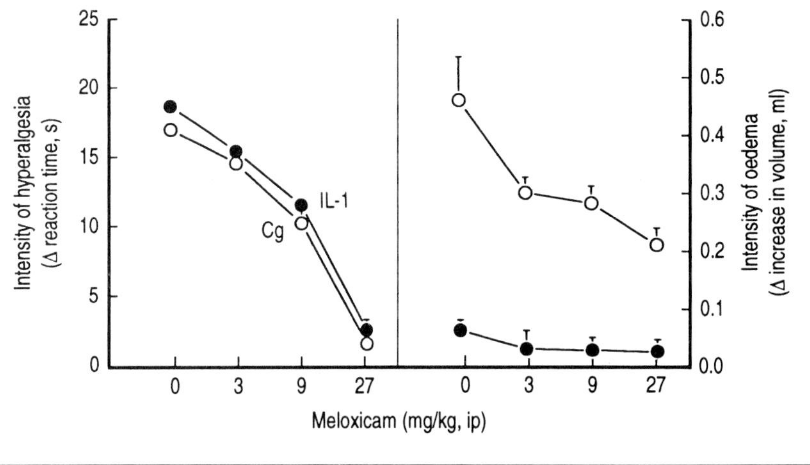

Figure 1   Dose-dependent effect of intraperitoneal meloxican upon the hyperalgesia and oedema induced by carrageenan and IL-1. Hyperalgesia was measured using the rat paw pressure test, a modification of the Randall–Selitto test, in which a constant pressure of 20 mmHg is applied to the rat paw and discontinued (reaction time) when the animal exhibits a freezing reaction[26]. The intensity of hyperalgesia was quantified as the difference in the reaction times (Δ reaction time) obtained by subtracting the value measured 3 h after administration of the hyperalgesic substances from the control reaction time measured prior to the administration of the hyperalgesic substance. The oedema was measured plethysmographically. Carrageenan (100 μg/paw) and IL-1 (0.5 pg/paw) were injected intraplantarly. Data are mean ± SEM of five animals per group

If the activation of PLA_2 constitutes, as generally assumed, the major rate limiting factor in the production of prostaglandins, intraplantar administration of arachidonic acid should cause hyperalgesia. The results shown in Figure 2 clearly disprove this concept. Arachidonic acid per se does not produce hyperalgesia, but potentiates that caused by carrageenan or IL-1β. It must be pointed out that in this model, carrageenan hyperalgesia depends on the release of IL-1β[20]. This cytokine induces COX-2 expression in many biological systems and carrageenan has been shown to cause induction of COX-2 in inflamed paws[6]. Figure 2 also illustrates that arachidonic acid does not potentiate the direct hyperalgesic effect of PGE_2 or of IL-8, which is known to cause hyperalgesia by the release of sympathetic amines[21]. These results are in accord with the concept that a COX is induced and activated during inflammatory reactions.

One of the characteristics of most inducible enzymes is the ability of cortico-steroids to inhibit their induction. Recently we demonstrated that the hyperalgesic effects of bradykinin, TNFα and IL-1β were inhibited by corticosteroids, and further, that this inhibition was abolished by pretreatment of the animals with anti-lipocortin-1 antibodies. The analgesic effect of corticosteroids was mimicked by treatment of

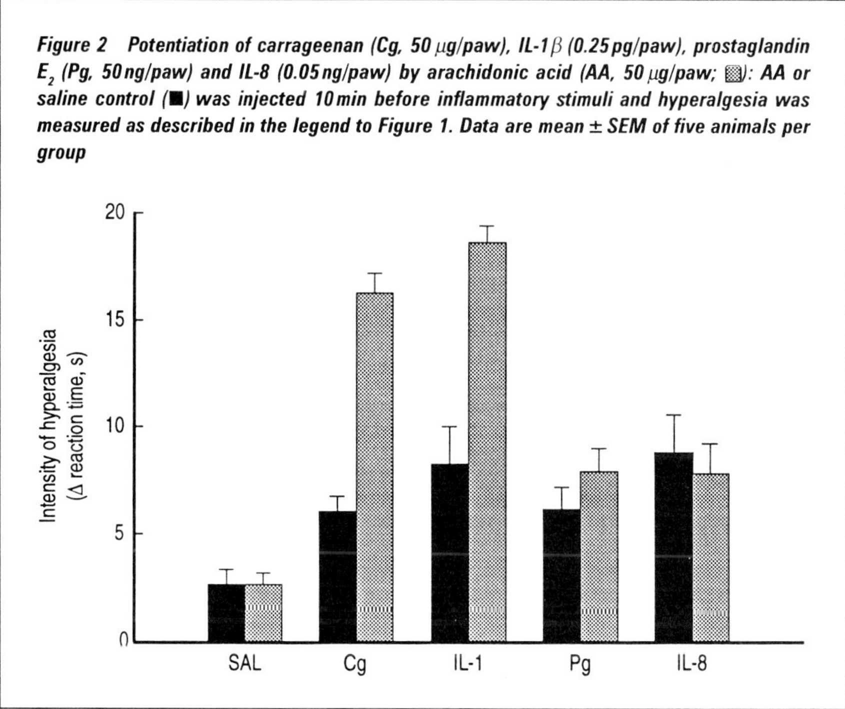

Figure 2 *Potentiation of carrageenan (Cg, 50 μg/paw), IL-1β (0.25 pg/paw), prostaglandin E_2 (Pg, 50 ng/paw) and IL-8 (0.05 ng/paw) by arachidonic acid (AA, 50 μg/paw; ▨): AA or saline control (■) was injected 10 min before inflammatory stimuli and hyperalgesia was measured as described in the legend to Figure 1. Data are mean ± SEM of five animals per group*

the paws with the lipocortin-1(2–26) fragment (unpublished results). In view of the absence of a hyperalgesic effect of arachidonic acid in normal paws it seems reasonable to suggest that the analgesic effect of corticosteroids, in addition to the blockade of the release of pro-inflammatory cytokines, also results from a blockade of the induction of an inducible COX. Our results indicate that the analgesic effect of corticosteroids in vivo is due to inhibition of cytokine release and possibly also to the blockade of the activation of COX-2 by IL-1β. COX-2 induction by an inflammatory stimulus has been described in the rat paw[6]. This suggestion is in line with the observation that the modulation of IL-8-induced COX-2 expression by corticosteroids is an important process in the inflammation of synovial tissues seen in patients with rheumatoid arthritis[25].

Figure 3 shows that the potentiation of IL-1- or carrageenan-induced hyperalgesia by arachidonic acid is significantly inhibited by meloxican. This is in line with the assumption that meloxican acts by inhibiting an inducible COX with the characteristics of COX 2.

CONCLUSION

Experimental evidence gained from gene disruptions in mice, which suggests that COX-1 rather than the inducible COX-2 is important for the inflammatory response,

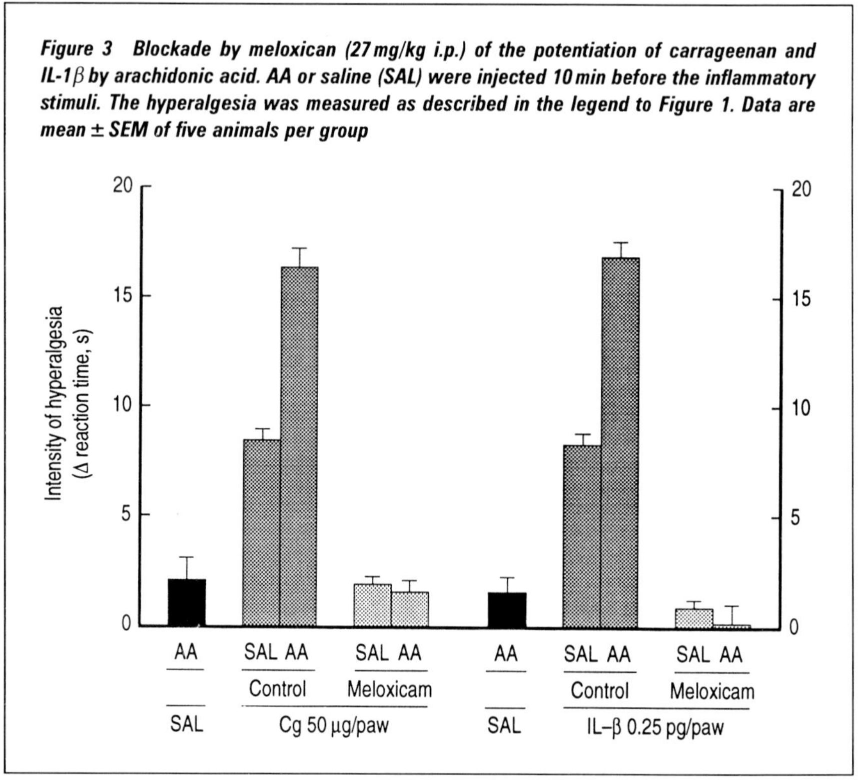

Figure 3 *Blockade by meloxican (27 mg/kg i.p.) of the potentiation of carrageenan and IL-1β by arachidonic acid. AA or saline (SAL) were injected 10 min before the inflammatory stimuli. The hyperalgesia was measured as described in the legend to Figure 1. Data are mean ± SEM of five animals per group*

contradicts the observations described here. Inhibition of an inducible COX significantly contributes to the analgesia and attenuation of oedema produced in rats by meloxican, a preferential inhibitor of the COX-2 enzyme.

References

1. Xie W, Robertson DL, Simmons DL. Mitogen-inducible prostaglandin G/H synthase: a new target for nonsteroidal antiinflammatory drugs. Drug Dev Res. 1992;25:249–65.
2. Grosman CJ, Wiesman J, Lucas FS, Trevethick, Birch PJ. Inhibition of constitutive and inducible cyclooxygenase activity in human platelets and mononuclear cells by NSAIDs and Cox 2 inhibitors. Inflamm Res. 1995;44:253–7.
3. Langenbach R, Morham SG, Tiano HF et al. Prostaglandin synthase 1 gene disruption in mice reduces arachidonic acid-induced inflammation and indomethacin-induced gastric ulceration. Cell. 1995;83:483–92.
4. Morham SG, Langenbach R, Loftin CD et al. Prostaglandin synthase 2 gene disruption causes severe renal pathology in the mouse. Cell. 1995;83:473–82.
5. Dinchuk JE, Car BD, Focht RJ et al. Renal abnormalities and an altered inflammatory response in mice lacking cyclooxygenase II. Nature. 1995;378:406–9.
6. Seibert K, Zhang Y, Leahy K et al. Pharmacological and biochemical demonstration of the role of cyclooxygenase 2 in inflammation and pain. Proc Natl Acad Sci USA. 1994;91:12013–17.

7. Engehart G, Homma D, Schlegel K, Utzmann R, Schinizler C. Antiinflammatory, analgesic, antipyretic and related properties of meloxicam, a new non-steroidal anti-inflammatory agent with favourable gastrointestinal tolerance. Inflamm Res. 1995;44:423–33.
8. Ferreira SH. Prostaglandins, aspirin-like drugs and analgesia. Nature New Biol. 1972;240:200–3.
9. Ferreira SH. A classification of peripheral analgesics based upon their mode of action. In: M. Sandler, GM Collins, editors. Migraine: Spectrum of Ideas. Oxford: Oxford University Press, 1990;59–72.
10. McMahon SB, Koltzenburg M. Novel classes of nociceptors: beyond Sherrington. Trends Neurosci. 1990;13:199–201.
11. Ferreira SH, Nakamura M. Prostaglandin hyperalgesia, a cAMP/Ca^{++} dependent process. Prostaglandins. 1979;18:179–90.
12. Taiwo YO, Bjerknes LK, Goetzl EJ, Levine JD. Mediation of primary afferent peripheral hyperalgesia by the cAMP second messenger system. Neuroscience. 1989;32:577–80.
13. Follenfant RL, Nakamura M, Garland LG. Sustained hyperalgesia in rats evoked by the protein kinase inhibitor H-7. Br J Pharmacol. 1990;99:289P.
14. Ferreira SH, Lorenzetti BB. Glutamate spinal retrograde sensitization of primary sensory neurons associated with nociception. Neuropharmacology. 1994;33:1479–85.
15. Duarte IDG, Lorenzetti BB, Ferreira SH. Peripheral analgesia and activation of the nitric oxide-cyclic GMP pathway. Eur J Pharmacol. 1990;186:289–93.
16. Ferreira SH, Duarte IDG, Lorenzetti BB. The molecular mechanism of action of peripheral morphine analgesia: stimulation of cGMP system via nitric oxide release. Eur J Pharmacol. 1991;201:121.
17. Duarte IDG, Lorenzetti BB, Ferreira SH. Acetylcholine induces peripheral analgesia by release of nitric oxide. In: S. Moncada, EA Higgs, editors. Nitric oxide from L-arginine: a bioregulatory system. Amsterdam: Elsevier Science Publishers, 1990;165–70.
18. Duarte IDG, Santos IR, Lorenzetti BB, Ferreira SH. Analgesia by direct antagonism of nociceptor sensitization involves the arginine-nitric oxide-cGMP pathway. Eur J Pharmacol. 1992;217:225–7.
19. Ferreira SH. Are macrophages the body's alarm cells? Agents Actions. 1980;10:229–30.
20. Ferreira SH, Lorenzetti BB, Bristow AF, Poole S. Interleukin-1β as a potent hyperalgesic agent antagonized by a tripeptide analogue. Nature. 1988;334:698–700.
21. Cunha FQ, Lorenzetti BB, Poole S, Ferreira SH. Interleukin 8 as a mediator of sympathetic pain. Br J Pharmacol. 1991;104:765–7.
22. Cunha FQ, Poole S, Lorenzetti BB, Ferreira SH. The pivotal role of tumour necrosis factor α in the development of inflammatory hyperalgesia. Br J Pharmacol. 1992;107:660–4.
23. Ferreira SH, Lorenzetti BB, Poole S, McMahon SB, Koltzenburg M. Bradykinin initiates cytokine-mediated inflammatory hyperalgesia. Br J Pharmacol. 1993;110:1227–31.
24. Li JJ, Anderson GD, Burton EG et al. 1,2-Diarylcyclopentenes as selective cyclooxygenase-2 inhibitors and orally active anti-inflammatory agents. J Med Chem. 1995;38:4570–8.
25. Crofford LJ, Wilder RL, Ristimaki AP et al. Cyclooxygenase-1 and -2 expression in rheumatoid synovial tissues. Effects of interleukin-1 beta, phorbol ester, and corticosteroids. J Clin Invest. 1994;93:1095–101.
26. Ferreira SH, Lorenzetti BB, Correa FM. Central and peripheral antialgesic action of aspirin-like drugs. Eur J Pharmacol. 1978;53:39–48.

5 Brain COX-2 in experimental models of epilepsy and stroke: signalling pathways leading to enhanced expression

N. G. BAZAN, V. M. MARCHESELLI, G. ALLAN,
K. VAN METER and J. P. MOISES

The response of the brain to ischaemia and seizures initially includes membrane depolarization, enhanced accumulation of phospholipid degradation products such as arachidonic acid[1], diacylglycerols[1] and platelet-activating factor (PAF)[2], increased glutamate release, and elevation of intracellular free calcium levels. Phospholipase activation and the release of bioactive lipids from membrane phospholipid pools represent part of an intrinsic neural inflammatory response in which first and second messengers such as PAF and arachidonic acid metabolites become injury signals in repeated seizures (status epilepticus) and ischaemia–reperfusion, thus promoting brain damage[3]. PAF is a transcriptional activator of COX-2[4], and is thus potentially part of a bioactive lipid cascade in which the early release of PAF gives rise to the delayed accumulation of prostaglandins, prostacyclin and thromboxanes. BN 50730, an intracellular PAF antagonist[5], blocks PAF-induced COX-2 expression. We therefore tested the effectiveness of BN 50730 in blocking induction of COX-2 mRNA and protein expression in vivo. The two models used were focal cerebral ischaemia using the suture model of middle cerebral artery occlusion (MCAO), and kainic acid (KA)-induced epileptogenesis. In focal cerebral ischaemia, the region of partially compromised tissue surrounding the central infarct, known as the penumbra, can potentially be salvaged; it is thus an important target for drugs that could limit neuronal damage. Cerebral ischaemia and ischaemia–reperfusion induced increases in COX-2 levels in the ischaemic core and penumbra, in agreement with a recent study[6]. A single intra-cerebroventricular injection of BN 50730, delivered prior to the start of ischaemia, inhibited COX-2 induction. NFκB, GAS/ISRE, AP2 and *zif-268* have been tentatively identified as transcription factors involved in the induction of COX-2 in hippocampus. Their DNA binding activities increased during MCAO and KA-induced seizures, but not when animals were pretreated with BN 50730.

In KA induced epileptogenesis, COX-2 accumulates mainly in the hippocampus, as a result of transcriptional activation rather than changes in mRNA stability. Induction of COX-2 expression in this model involves the NMDA receptor, since it is inhibited by the NMDA receptor antagonist MK801[7]. COX-2 expression has been shown to be induced during synaptic plasticity responses[8], and thus over-expression may initiate pathological forms of neuroplasticity in epileptogenesis. The use of selective COX-2 inhibitors therefore represents a novel approach to controlling the neural inflammatory response in cerebral ischaemia and seizures.

INDUCIBLE PROSTAGLANDIN SYNTHASE IN BRAIN

The conversion of arachidonic acid into biologically-active prostaglandins (PG), prostacyclin and thromboxanes proceeds through an initial, rate-limiting step catalysed by prostaglandin synthase (PGS, also known as prostaglandin endoperoxide synthase, PGH synthase, cyclooxygenase, COX, 5Z, 8Z, 11Z, 14Z-icosa-5, 8, 11, 14-tetraenoate, hydrogen donor:oxygen oxide reductase; EC1.14.99.1). The enzyme catalyses two distinct reactions, cyclooxygenation of the fatty acid to the unstable intermediate PGG_2 and the subsequent peroxidation to yield PGH_2. There are two isoforms of PG synthase, COX-1 and the more recently discovered COX-2, which are structurally homologous and catalyse the same reaction with similar kinetics. They are, however, encoded by distinct genes and have very different patterns of expression. COX-1 is constitutively expressed in a wide range of tissues and gene expression does not appear to be subject to regulation other than during development. By contrast, basal expression of COX-2 is limited to a few specialized tissues, but is rapidly and transiently induced in many cells and tissues in response to mitogens and cytokines. COX-2 is, in fact, an immediate-early gene, i.e. one that exhibits stimulus-evoked transient expression in the absence of de novo protein synthesis. Glucocorticoids inhibit COX-2 induction in most cell types and, in vivo, are thought to exert a tonic regulation on COX-2 expression[9]. COX-2 is, in fact, only one of a whole series of genes the induction of which is attenuated by glucocorticoids. These include the inducible form of nitric oxide synthase, various chemokines, growth regulators and proteins with as yet unknown function. The common motif among the known glucocorticoid-attenuated response genes (GARGs)[10] is an involvement in extracellular communication and modulation of inflammation and mitogenesis. The physiological significance of this action of glucocorticoids is thought to be that adrenocortical activity exerts a tonic regulation on these aspects of development and inflammation. COX-2 has been cloned independently from a number of sources, including a TPA-inducible gene in Swiss 3T3 fibroblasts[11], a growth factor-induced gene in chick fibroblasts[12], and a glucocorticoid-regulated gene PG synthase in mouse fibroblasts[13].

The brain is one of the few sites in which COX-2 is expressed constitutively, albeit at lower levels than in the induced state. Significantly, given that glia are thought to be the major endogenous inflammatory cells in the brain, COX-2 expression is found mainly in neurones[8,14]. COX-2 mRNA is found in discrete cellular populations throughout the forebrain of the rat, and is enriched in the cerebral cortex and hippocampus. Expression is rapidly and transiently increased in response to seizures and NMDA-dependent synaptic activity, while basal expression in the developing and adult brain appears to be regulated by synaptic activity. Specifically, detectable basal expression in the developing rat brain is noted from postnatal day 5 onwards, a period of massive synaptic plasticity and developmental changes. The inducibility of COX-2 expression in response to synaptic stimuli implies a role in neuronal plasticity.

COX-2 IS INDUCED IN NEUROTRAUMA: A ROLE FOR PAF

COX-2 has been shown to be induced in the brain in two experimental models of trauma, KA-induced seizures[15] and vasogenic oedema[16]. Treatment with KA induced a generalized up-regulation of COX-2 mRNA levels in the forebrain, but expression persisted for much longer in brain regions known to be vulnerable to kainate-induced neuronal necrosis. In the oedema model, expression of COX-2 mRNA and protein was up-regulated by the insult. Pretreatment of the animals with the PAF antagonist BN 50730 attenuated COX-2 induction and also reduced the magnitude of cerebral oedema. As in other tissues and cells, peak expression of COX-2 mRNA and protein is delayed compared with that of immediate-early gene transcription factors (e.g. c-Fos, *zif-268*). However, unlike in vitro models, the expression of the protein remains above basal levels even after 24h. Although it could be argued that BN 50730 inhibition of COX-2 expression was not necessarily related to oedema reduction, dexamethasone pretreatment also reduced both COX-2 induction and cerebral oedema.

A 'PAF-RESPONSIVE ELEMENT' IN THE COX-2 PROMOTER

In vitro studies on rat COX-2 promoter-driven reporter gene expression demonstrate a PAF-responsive region[4]. When constructs are transfected into cells using the calcium phosphate-calcium co-precipitation procedure in the presence of retinoic acid, the PAF-induced expression of the reporter driven by the proximal 371 bp of the mouse COX-2 promoter is dose-dependent (1–50nmol). There is also activity from a 963 bp promoter fragment, although this is less, which suggests that inhibitory sequences reside upstream from −371bp. The effect is rapid, with some activity after as little as 15–45 min of incubation with the ligands, suggesting that pre-existing transcription factors are involved. Preincubation of the cells with BN 50730 provides further evidence that this effect is a specific receptor-mediated phenomenon. The use of constructs with 5′ deletions of this promoter narrows down the main 'PAF-responsive' region of the promoter to between −371 and −300; deletion of this region lowers PAF induction from 31 times to 4.1 times control levels.

PAF RECEPTORS AND SIGNAL TRANSDUCTION

The PAF receptor has a predicted secondary amino structure characteristic of the rhodopsin-type receptor super-family, i.e. G protein-coupled cell-surface receptors with seven membrane-spanning domains[17-19]. Analysis of the PAF receptor gene structure shows two different transcription start sites contained in two distinct 5′ non-coding exons[20]. When alternatively spliced to a common exon containing the entire coding sequence, the result is the expression of two different transcripts (types 1 and 2) that contain the identical coding sequence but differ in their 5′ untranslated leader sequences. The leader sequences of types 1 and 2 both contain consensus binding sequences for the transcription factors NFκB and Sp-1, but type 2 alone contains additional binding sequences for AP-1 and AP-2. The transcripts show differential expression, types 1 and 2 being expressed in heart, spleen and kidney, and type 1 alone in brain and peripheral leukocytes. The significance of two distinct transcripts has not been fully assessed. One recent study showed that retinoic acid and thyroid hormone regulate PAF receptor expression, but only in tissues in which the type 2 mRNA is expressed[21].

Various biochemical studies suggest that the primary mode of signal transduction for the PAF receptor is via a G protein-linked inositol phospholipid-specific phospholipase C[22,23]. This couples PAF receptor activation with the classical bifurcating signal transduction pathway in which diacylglycerol activates protein kinase C and inositol trisphosphate mobilizes intracellular calcium stores. PAF treatment of hippocampal neurones in culture elicits intracellular calcium fluxes, with dynamics characteristic of release from intracellular stores[24]. PAF receptor activation has also been shown to stimulate the mitogen-associated protein (MAP) kinase and related protein kinase cascades[25,26] and to down-regulate cyclic AMP formation[27]. In some neuronal cell lines, PAF can raise intracellular calcium in the presence of extracellular calcium, indicating the activation of cell-surface calcium channels[28].

PAF receptors have also been detected in rat cerebral cortex and hippocampus using ligand binding assays on cortical subcellular fractions[5,29]. These studies showed two different types of binding sites, one in synaptosomal membranes and another in microsomal membranes. The two sites differ in the kinetics of [^{3}H]PAF binding and microsomal membranes display cold-ligand displacement kinetics characteristic of two binding sites. The synaptosomal and microsomal sites also differ in their sensitivity to two distinct types of PAF receptor antagonist, which in turn appear to influence different aspects of PAF action in the CNS. BN 52021, a terpenoid extracted from the leaf of the *Ginkgo biloba* tree, binds preferentially to the synaptosomal site whereas the synthetic hetrazepine BN 50730 shows specificity for the microsomal sites[5,29]. The BN 52021-sensitive PAF binding site appears to correspond to the cloned PAF receptor and to mediate the effects of PAF at the synapse. This antagonist selectively inhibits glutamate release from hippocampal neurones[30], perforant path LTP in hippocampal slices[31] and PAF-induced enhancement of memory tasks related to structures in the limbic system[32]. The BN 50730-sensitive site has yet to be isolated and there is no indication whether this represents an isoform of the cell-surface receptor, or a completely novel type of PAF receptor. There is also no indication yet as to which cell type(s) in the CNS express this form of PAF receptor. Thus far, the BN 50730-sensitive receptor has been linked with PAF-mediated effects on gene expression in the CNS. For example, BN 50730, but not BN 52021, inhibits PAF- and neurotrauma-induced expression of the immediate-early genes *zif-268, c-fos* and COX-2[5,16].

COX-2 INHIBITION: A NEW STRATEGY FOR NEUROPROTECTION

The effects of cerebral ischaemia on excitable membranes, as well as other neurochemical and functional changes, are reflected in the accumulation of membrane-derived lipid second messengers. This accumulation in the synapse during injury represents an overactivation of processes that regulate normal synaptic function. It may play a central role in various pathways leading to brain damage. However, some of these mediators may also activate cellular routes leading to plasticity responses and repair.

Different neurones maintain networks of complex interactions between themselves and other cell types. There are, however, predominant pathways. First, some signals converge to promote excitotoxicity by enhancing glutamate release through PAF, and/ or other mediators, acting on the presynaptic terminal. There is an overactivation of postsynaptic glutamate receptors, a sharp elevation of intracellular calcium levels and overproduction of membrane phospholipid-derived second messengers. An early indicator of the degree of cerebral ischaemia is the accumulation of free poly-unsaturated fatty acids. Membrane phospholipid breakdown, reperfusion and other factors contribute to the initiation of oxygen radical reactions that include lipid peroxidation and secondary decrease in blood flow. Moreover, by damaging structural and functional components of the cell, oxidative stress plays a major role in limiting neural cell survival in stroke. Second, there are multiple mediators of the inflammatory response generated. Third, some neurones die early after a cerebrovascular insult, some recover, while others exhibit delayed apoptotic death as a consequence of some initial events. Lastly, it is likely that there are signals that activate plasticity and repair pathways that, in turn, lead to the re-establishment of synaptic circuitry.

Following stroke, there is sometimes remarkable recovery weeks after an initially severe neurological impairment. This may be due to resolution of the injury–inflammatory condition, active neural plasticity that re-establishes some damaged synaptic circuitry, or remodelling of extracellular matrix components important for blood–brain barrier function and for intercellular relationships. Some membrane-derived lipid second messengers generated in the acute response to injury may participate in the coupling of injury either with repair/regenerative responses, or with cell death via the activation of gene cascades, as discussed above.

Several physiological mediators in the nervous system may also play roles in patho-logical conditions. Glutamate, an excitatory amino acid, is by far the most abundant neurotransmitter in the mammalian brain and plays a critical role in developmental plasticity, memory formation, etc. However, in neurotrauma and some neuro-degenerative diseases, glutamate accumulates to abnormally high levels, making it a critical effector of neuronal damage. Other mediators, such as interleukin-1 and, perhaps, amyloid peptide, also co-exist with neural cells under physiological conditions but, like PAF, may engage in abnormal actions in diseases when overproduced. Although PAF is most often referred to as a mediator of the inflammatory and immune responses and of cell injury, low PAF concentrations elicit sprouting in PC12 cells. At high concentrations, neuropathological changes occur. The presynaptic PAF binding site, linked to glutamate release, is a target through which PAF participates in excitotoxicity. However, the same presynaptic site involves PAF as a potential retrograde messenger in long-term potentiation and synaptic plasticity.

The inducible prostaglandin synthase gene (COX-2) represents a link between ischaemia-generated PAF and the cyclooxygenation of arachidonic acid. Prostaglandin synthase isoenzymes in the brain, and their physiological significance and pathological roles, are only beginning to be studied. Experimental evidence thus far has shown protective effects of COX-2 inhibition at the blood–brain barrier. Whereas prolonged COX-2 up-regulation has been spatially correlated to regions vulnerable to kainate-induced necrosis, the direct consequences on the progression of neuronal damage have yet to be assessed. Because PAF synthesis is also activated by glutamate/NMDA receptor interaction, it is possible that the induction of prostaglandin synthase in brain may open a pathway involved in modulation of synaptic function. Inducible prostaglandin synthase in neurotraumatic injury has thus far only been shown to be involved in events at the blood–brain barrier, and presumably represents actions on the vascular endothelium. The pathophysiological actions of prostanoids generated by COX-2 induction within the brain (i.e. on neurones and glia) are currently under investigation.

Acknowledgement

This work is supported by National Institutes of Health grant NS23002.

References

1. Bazan NG. Effects of ischemia and electroconvulsive shock on free fatty acid pool in the brain. Biochim Biophys Acta. 1970;218:1–10.
2. Kumar R, Harvey S, Kester N, Hanahan D, Olsen M. Production and effects of platelet-activating factor in the rat brain. Biochim Biophys Acta. 1988;963:375–83.
3. Bazan NG. Inflammation: A signal terminator. Nature. 1995;374:501–2.
4. Bazan NG, Fletcher BS, Herschman HR, Mukherjee PK. Platelet-activating factor and retinoic acid synergistically activate the inducible prostaglandin synthase gene. Proc Natl Acad Sci USA. 1994;91:5252–6.
5. Marcheselli VL, Bazan NG. Platelet-activating factor is a messenger in the electroconvulsive shock-induced transcriptional activation of c-*fos* and *zif*-268 in hippocampus. J Neurosci Res. 1994;37:54–61.
6. Planas AM, Soriano MA, Rodriguez-Farre E, Ferrer I. Induction of cyclooxygenase-2 mRNA and protein following transient focal ischemia in the rat brain. Neurosci Lett. 1995;200:187–90.
7. Adams J, Collaco-Moraes Y, de Belleroche J. Cyclooxygenase-2 induction in cerebral cortex: an intracellular response to synaptic excitation. J Neurochem. 1996;66:6–13.
8. Yamagata K, Andreasson KI, Kaufmann WE, Barnes CA, Worley PF. Expression of a mitogen-inducible cyclooxygenase in brain neurons: regulation by synaptic activity and glucocorticoids. Neuron. 1993;11:371–86.
9. Herschman HR. Regulation of prostaglandin synthase-1 and prostaglandin synthase-2. Cancer Metastasis Rev. 1994;13:241–56.
10. Smith JB, Herschman HR. Glucocorticoid-attenuated response genes encode intercellular mediators, including a new C-X-C chemokine. J Biol Chem. 1995;270:16756–65.
11. Kujubu DA, Fletcher BS, Varnum BC, Lim RW, Herschman HR. TIS10, a phorbol ester tumor promoter-inducible mRNA from Swiss 3T3 cells, encodes a novel prostaglandin synthase/cyclo-oxygenase homologue. J Biol Chem. 1991;266:12866–72.
12. Xie W, Chipman JG, Robertson DL, Simmons DL. Expression of a mitogen-responsive gene encoding prostaglandin synthase is regulated by mRNA splicing. Proc Natl Acad Sci USA. 1991;88:2692–6.
13. O'Banion MK, Winn VP, Yang DA. c-DNA cloning and functional activity of a glucocorticoid-regulated inflammatory cyclooxygenase. Proc Natl Acad Sci USA. 1992;89:4888–92.
14. Breder CD, DeWitt D, Kraig RP. Characterization of inducible cyclooxygenase in rat brain. J Comp Neurol. 1995;355:296–315.
15. Chen J, Marxh T, Zhang JS, Graham SH. Expression of cyclo-oxygenase 2 in rat brain following kainate treatment. NeuroReport. 1995;6:245–8.
16. Bazan NG, Marcheselli VL, Allan G. An inhibitor of injury-induced COX-2 transcriptional activation elicits neuroprotection in a brain damage model. In: J Vane, J Botting, R. Botting (editors) Improved Non-Steroid Anti-Inflammatory Drugs: COX-2 Enzyme Inhibitors. 9th edn. Lancaster: Kluwer Academic Publishers. 1996:145–66.
17. Honda Z, Nakamura M, Miki I et al. Cloning by functional expression of platelet-activating factor receptor from guinea-pig lung. Nature. 1991;394:342–6.

18. Kunz D, Gerard NP, Gerard C. The human leukocyte PAF receptor. cDNA cloning, cell surface expression and construction of a novel epitope-bearing analog. J Biol Chem. 1992;267:9101–6.
19. Sugimoto T, Tsuchimochi H, McGregor CG, Mutoh H, Shimizu T, Kurachi Y. Molecular cloning and characterization of the platelet-activating factor receptor from human heart. Biochem Biophys Res Commun. 1992;189:617–24.
20. Mutoh H, Bito H, Minami M et al. Two different promoters direct expression of two distinct forms of mRNA of human platelet-activating factor receptor. FEBS Lett. 1993;322:129–34.
21. Mutoh H, Jukuda T, Kitamaoto T et al. Tissue-specific response of the human platelet-activating factor receptor gene to retinoic acid and thyroid hormone by alternative promoter usage. Proc Natl Acad Sci USA. 1996;93:774–9.
22. Ali H, Richardson RM, Tomhave ED, DuBose RA, Haribabu B, Snyderman R. Regulation of stably transfected platelet activating factor receptor in RBL-2H3 cells. Role of multiple G proteins and receptor phosphorylation. J Biol Chem. 1994;269:24557–63.
23. Honda Z, Takano T, Hirose N et al. Gq pathway desensitizes chemotactic receptor-induced calcium signaling via inositol trisphosphate receptor down-regulation. J Biol Chem. 1995;270:2840–4.
24. Bito H, Nakamura M, Honda A et al. Platelet-activating factor (PAF) receptor in rat brain: PAF mobilizes intracellular Ca^{2+} in hippocampal neurons. Neuron. 1992;9:1–10.
25. Hanahan DJ. Platelet-activating factor: a novel lipid agonist. Curr Topics Cell Reg. 1992;33:65–78.
26. Kuruvilla A, Pielop C, Shearer WT. Platelet-activating factor induces the tyrosine phosphorylation and activation of phospholipase C-gamma 1, Fyn and Lyn kinases, and phosphatidylinositol 3-kinase in a human B cell line. J Immunol. 1994;153:5433–42.
27. Kester M, Thomas CP, Wang J, Dunn MJ. Platelet-activating factor stimulates multiple signaling pathways in cultured rat mesangial cells. J Cell Physiol. 1992;153:244–55.
28. Kornecki E, Ehrlich YH. Neuroregulatory and neuropathological actions of the ether-phospholipid platelet-activating factor. Science. 1988;240:1792–4.
29. Marcheselli VL, Rossowska M, Domingo MT, Braquet P, Bazan NG. Distinct platelet-activating factor binding sites in synaptic endings and in intracellular membranes of rat cerebral cortex. J Biol Chem. 1990;265:9140–5.
30. Clark GD, Happel LT, Zorumski CF, Bazan NG. Enhancement of hippocampal excitatory synaptic transmission by platelet-activating factor. Neuron. 1992;9:1211–16.
31. Kato K, Clark GD, Bazan NG, Zorumski CF. Platelet-activating factor as a potential retrograde messenger in CA1 hippocampal long-term potentiation. Nature. 1994;367:179–82.
32. Izquierdo I, Fin C, Schmitz PK et al. Memory enhancement by intrahippocampal, intraamygdala, or intraentorhinal infusion of platelet-activating factor measured in an inhibitory avoidance task. Proc Natl Acad Sci USA. 1995;92:5047–51.

6 New highly selective cyclooxygenase-2 inhibitors

A. W. FORD-HUTCHINSON

It has been recognized recently that cyclooxygenase (prostaglandin G/H-synthase) exists in two isoforms which have been termed COX-1 (constitutive enzyme) and COX-2 (inducible enzyme)[1,2]. COX-1 has been cloned from a number of sources including mouse, man and sheep[3-7]. COX-2 was originally identified as a v-*src*-inducible gene product in chicken fibroblasts and as a phorbol ester-inducible early gene product in murine 3T3 cells[8,9]. These proteins were recognized as novel cyclooxygenases by their homology with COX-1. The human COX-2 cDNA was subsequently cloned and shown to have 64% overall amino acid sequence identity to human COX-1[10]. There are a number of similarities between the two isoforms: both proteins contain a signal peptide sequence, a putative membrane anchoring domain, a conserved active site, an aspirin acetylation site and a C-terminal STEL sequence which may be responsible for retaining the protein in the endoplasmic reticulum. The main significant difference between COX-2 and COX-1 is that COX-2 can be induced transiently over a >50-fold range by a variety of agents, including cytokines, phorbol esters, hormones, serum and lipopolysaccharide. This induction can be inhibited by glucocorticoids. As might be anticipated, the structures of the 5′ region of the genes are very different between the two enzymes[2].

It is well established that the mechanism of action of non-steroid anti-inflammatory drugs (NSAIDs) involves inhibition of cyclooxygenase[11,12]. In addition, inhibition of the production of prostaglandins explains the anti-inflammatory, analgesic and anti-pyretic activity of these compounds, as well as their ability to inhibit hormone-induced uterine contractions and the growth of certain types of cancer. It is also clear that NSAIDs have mechanism-based side effects, including gastrointestinal lesions, effects on renal function in compromised individuals, increases in bleeding time, induction of asthma and prolongation of gestation and labour. Thus, it is clear that prostanoids have both physiological and pathological effects. The hypothesis behind the development of selective COX-2 inhibitors is that the therapeutic usefulness of NSAIDs will be largely due to inhibition of inducible COX-2, while the side effect profile will be largely due to inhibition of COX-1[1,13]. None of the conventional NSAIDs currently available in North America show a significant degree of selectivity for either COX-1 or COX-2.

DEVELOPMENT OF COX-2 INHIBITORS

There are two general classes of COX-2 inhibitors (Figure 1). These include sulphonamides, as exemplified by the Taisho compound NS-398[14] and flosulide[15] and

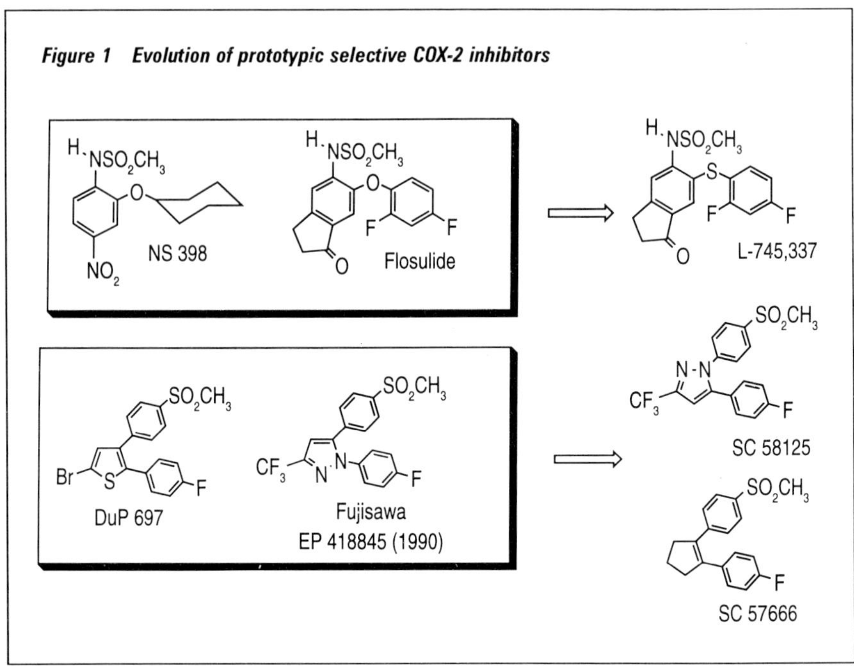

tricyclic methylsulphone derivatives, as exemplified by the prototypic compound DuP-697[16]. These compounds have led to the synthesis of a derivative of flosulide, L-745,337, which has been used in animal studies to test the COX-2 hypothesis[17–19], as well as a number of tricyclic methylsulphones with improved selectivity for COX-2[20–23].

In order to provide a rational basis for designing selective COX-2 inhibitors, crystal structures of cyclooxygenase isozymes have been obtained. The three-dimensional structure of ovine COX-1, crystallized as a homodimer, reveals that the mature enzyme is composed of three distinct domains: an epidermal growth factor-like module, a membrane-binding motif containing four α-helices and a catalytic domain[24]. The latter is a globular structure containing the cyclooxygenase active site at the end of the long, hydrophobic channel, the opening of which is circumscribed by the four membrane-associated α-helices. The non-selective NSAID flurbiprofen binds directly in the cyclooxygenase active site, the carboxylic acid group of the drug interacting with an arginine (residue 120) proximal to the membrane-associating α-helices of COX-1. Although COX-1 and COX-2 show an overall 61% amino acid identity, the residues surrounding the active site are almost entirely conserved and crystal structures and modelling studies predict that these differences should not result in large changes in the substrate binding pocket. To study the functional role of Arg-120 in COX-1, this residue was mutated to glutamic acid and expressed in a vaccinia virus system[25]. This human COX-1 (Arg-120$\rightarrow$Glu) showed a 20-fold reduction in specific activity and 100-fold increase in the apparent k_m for arachidonic acid. This mutation dramatically affected the ability of acidic NSAIDs to inhibit the enzyme. Indomethacin, flurbiprofen and ketoprofen showed no inhibitory activity against the mutated enzyme and diclofenac and meclofenamic acid were 50- to 100-fold less potent as inhibitors. In contrast, the non-acidic tricyclic compounds (DuP-697 and a dibromo-sulphonamide analogue of DuP-697) were both more potent inhibitors of the mutant enzyme than the wild type enzyme. Such data indicate the importance of the Arg-120 residue of COX-1 in the interaction of the enzyme with both arachidonic acid and conventional acidic NSAIDs, and also suggest that non-acidic selective COX-2 inhibitors, particularly of the tricyclic series containing a methylsulphone moiety, bind in a different fashion to the enzyme.

MECHANISTIC STUDIES ON COX-2 INHIBITORS

Inhibition of COX-1 or COX-2 by potent inhibitors is time-dependent in both cell-free and whole cell assays. Upon mixing enzyme and inhibitor, the inhibition develops to its maximum level over a period ranging from minutes to hours. Increased inhibitor concentrations result in a faster inhibition. This behaviour is rationalized in terms of initial low affinity binding of the inhibitor in a rapidly reversible step, followed by a slower transition to a state in which the inhibitors are more tightly bound to the enzyme. This means that the fully developed time-dependent inhibition is only very slowly reversible. As inhibition of cyclooxygenase by most NSAIDs is believed to be competitive with substrate, increasing arachidonic acid concentrations will increase the time required for the development of maximal inhibition of a time-dependent inhibitor.

The implications of this time-dependent inhibition are that inhibition of the enzyme target in vivo can persist even after plasma levels of the inhibitor have fallen well below that required for inhibition. In this case the duration of action of the drug may be limited more by the rate of de novo synthesis of the cyclooxygenase than by the pharmacokinetic parameters of the drug itself. This type of behaviour, however, is a significant liability for the development of selective COX-2 inhibitors: rapid induction of COX-2 may result in the production of enzyme which is not exposed to inhibitor for a sufficient time before it begins acting upon a substrate. The enzyme might produce sufficient product before development of maximum inhibition, thus rendering the inhibition functionally ineffective.

Figure 2 shows the mechanism of action of selective COX-2 inhibitors on both COX-1 and COX-2[26,27]. Inhibition of COX-1 by selective COX-2 inhibitors is weak, but not time dependent: a selective COX-2 inhibitor will initially function as a relatively weak, rapidly reversible inhibitor of the enzyme. Maximum inhibition will develop over a period of time, depending on the degree of time-dependence of inhibition. Thus the selectivity of potent COX-2 inhibitors, which is only produced through this time-dependent interaction, will not be realized at early times after expression of COX-2. This will be particularly aggravated in acute inflammatory situations in which high arachidonic concentrations may be present, and which should result in an even lesser degree of functional selectivity. It is very difficult to estimate the extent to which these factors influence the in vivo selectivity and potency

Figure 2   Mechanism of action of selective COX-2 inhibitors. Selectivity for COX-2 over COX-1 is achieved by the time-dependent and essentially irreversible formation of the EI* complex

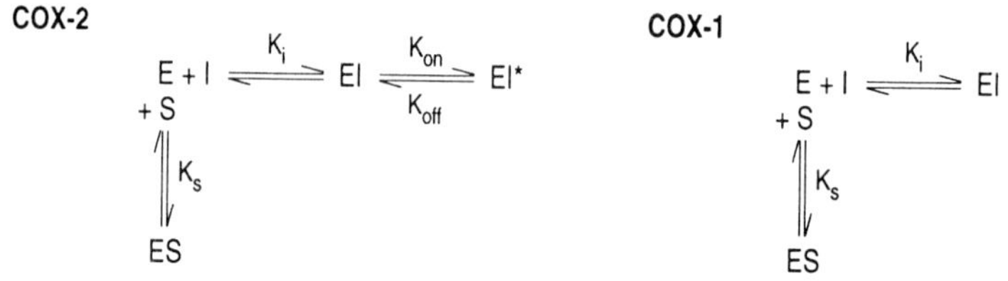

of selective COX-2 inhibitors, but such factors are clearly important. This mechanism explains the wide variety of IC_{50} values obtained with various inhibitors under different conditions of preincubation, substrate concentrations and enzyme concentrations, and strongly suggests that extremely high degrees of selectivity will be required to produce functional selectivity in vivo and hence reduction of COX-1-mediated side effects.

ANTI-INFLAMMATORY, ANALGESIC AND ANTI-PYRETIC ACTIVITIES OF COX-2 INHIBITORS

A key issue is whether selective COX-2 inhibitors will have equivalent anti-inflammatory, analgesic and anti-pyretic activity to mixed COX-1 and COX-2 inhibitors (conventional NSAIDs). Studies carried out with the prototypic COX-2 inhibitor L-745,337 and other related COX-2 inhibitors in animals have shown that these compounds produce similar reversals of pain and fever responses to those produced by indomethacin[17,18]. These compounds also showed anti-inflammatory activity similar to conventional NSAIDs in the rat carageenan paw oedema and the adjuvant arthritis models, which have been shown to be predictive of activity in man[18,22,23]. These results do not exclude the possibility that in certain acute situations prostaglandins may be released from constitutive COX-1 before induction of COX-2, and may contribute to early pain and inflammatory responses. It is also unclear whether the absence of mechanism-based side effects with COX-2 inhibitors will allow for higher dosing in man, leading to more complete suppression of prostaglandin production and hence to improved anti-inflammatory activity.

COX-2 INHIBITORS AND THEIR POTENTIAL FOR INDUCING GASTROINTESTINAL LESIONS

The use of NSAIDs has been estimated to result in 76 000 hospitalizations and 7600 deaths per year in the USA[28]. These observations indicate that prostaglandins play important physiological roles within the gastrointestinal tract, where they appear to be involved in numerous processes, including control of gastric acid secretion, mucus production and maintenance of mucosal integrity and blood flow[29–32]. In the lower gastrointestinal tract they appear to be involved in the modulation of colonic motility, electrolyte and water secretion and proliferative activity within the colon[30,33]. Prostaglandin may be produced from multiple cell types within the intestinal tract, including colonic and intestinal epithelial cells, immune cells in the lamina propria and subepithelial mesenchymal cells[34].

Since the discovery of COX-2, studies have attempted to assess the expression of both COX-1 and COX-2 in the gastrointestinal tract of human and various animal species. In general, ubiquitous expression of COX-1 protein has been observed in a variety of gastrointestinal tissues from several species, while expression of COX-2 proteins was absent from most gastrointestinal tissues examined[35,36]. Small amounts of COX-2 may be present in certain tissues, such as in rat caecum[36], consistent with observations that COX-2 proteins in rat intestinal epithelial cells can be stimulated with transforming growth factor-α. In contrast to the lack of expression of COX-2 in normal human intestinal tissues, significant levels of COX-2 have been observed in samples of colon cancer[35,37,38]. This has been interpreted as indicating that the protective effects of NSAIDs against colon cancer may be mediated by inhibition of COX-2.

Acute studies with various prototypic COX-2 inhibitors in animals seem to indicate that such compounds lack the gastric toxicity associated with NSAIDs. Rats and squirrel monkeys were given L-745,337 for 4–5 days, twice daily, with subsequent monitoring of gastrointestinal damage through the faecal excretion of $^{51}CrCl_3$. Dramatic differences were observed between the selective COX-2 inhibitor and conventional NSAIDs with regard to their potential for inducing leakage in the gastrointestinal tract[18], and this was interpreted to indicate that inhibition of COX-1 in the gastrointestinal tract is responsible for the gastrointestinal injury induced by NSAIDs. Surprisingly however, COX-1 deficient knockout mice are generally healthy, do not have spontaneous stomach ulcers and show less gastric ulceration than wild type mice after gavage with indomethacin[39]. The result can be interpreted in one of three ways. Either a compensatory mechanism may exist in COX-1 knockout mice to maintain gastric mucosal integrity in the absence of the constitutive enzyme, or the absence of COX-1 is not itself sufficient to cause stomach ulceration in mice. Stomach ulceration instead could be due to either inhibition of both COX-1 and COX-2 or another unrelated mechanism combined with inhibition of COX-1. These issues will have to be addressed in large scale, long term clinical trials of selective COX-2 inhibitors in man, with monitoring of the comparative rates of ulceration and intestinal permeability using a variety of methods. If COX 2 inhibitors are to be of value as novel, safer therapeutic agents then such trials will have to show a significant reduction in gastrointestinal lesions compared with conventional NSAIDs and such data should translate into reductions in the number of hospital admissions and deaths associated with the use of this class of agent.

COX-2 INHIBITORS AND PLATELET FUNCTION

Platelets have been reported to possess only COX-1: COX-2 protein cannot be detected by Western blot analysis. COX-2 inhibitors therefore have no effect on platelet thromboxane B_2 production and thus will have no effect on the aggregation of platelets induced by a variety of agents including collagen, ADP and thromboxane mimetics. These results indicate that selective COX-2 inhibitors will not increase bleeding times, unlike conventional NSAIDs, which are contraindicated in patients with gastrointestinal bleeding, coagulation disorders and other bleeding problems, as well as in patients prior to surgery or those taking anti-coagulants. Such restrictions may not be applicable to COX-2 selective compounds.

COX-2 INHIBITORS AND RENAL FUNCTION

Prostaglandins may have an important modulatory role in the kidney through their control of several renal events, including renin release, salt and water reabsorption, renal blood flow redistribution and the control of renal vascular resistance and glomerular filtration[40–42]. In patients with impaired kidney function, administration of NSAIDs induces a reduction in glomerular filtration rate, associated with water and sodium retention and a decrease in renal blood flow. These patients can be classified into two groups. First, there are those showing activation of systemic or renal vasoconstrictor systems (e.g. the sympathetic nervous system or angiotensin-II) including volume depletion, hypotension, congestive heart failure, hepatic cirrhosis with ascites, nephrotic syndrome, patent ductus arteriosus, etc. Second, there are those with diseases directly affecting the kidneys such as lupus nephritis and pyelonephritis. 'Unexpected' deterioration of renal function occurs most often in the former group.

COX-1 is abundantly expressed throughout the kidney. Regulation of COX-2 expression has been observed in kidneys in the macula densa following salt deprivation[43]. Similarly, pharmacological studies in the rabbit have shown that the increased or exaggerated prostaglandin production observed in hydronephrotic kidneys is attributable to COX-2, whereas the basal release of prostaglandins is attributable to COX-1[44]. These results suggest that prostaglandin production in the normal kidney is driven by the activity of COX-1, while kidneys subject to either inflammatory or other challenges can show induction of COX-2. Detailed studies will be required in man to determine whether selective COX-2 inhibitors will possess some or all of the renal side effects associated with conventional NSAIDs.

CONCLUSION

Preclinical data support the hypothesis that selective COX-2 inhibitors will have anti-inflammatory, analgesic and anti-pyretic activities comparable to those of conventional NSAIDs, with a substantial reduction in some of the side effects associated with this class of drugs, particularly induction of gastric lesions and effects on bleeding times. The effects of selective COX-2 inhibitors on kidney function in individuals with renal compromise are less clear. Mechanistic studies indicate that a high degree of selectivity for COX-2 will be required for effective functional selectivity in vivo. A number of highly selective COX-2 inhibitors have been synthesized and described in the patent literature and hopefully in the near future clinical data on such inhibitors will be available to help assess the validity of the hypothesis.

References

1. Smith WL, DeWitt DL. Biochemistry of prostaglandin endoperoxide H synthase-1 and synthase-2 and their differential susceptibility to nonsteroidal anti-inflammatory drugs. Semin Nephrol. 1995;15:179–94.
2. Herschman HR. Prostaglandin synthase-2. Biochim Biophys Acta. 1996;1299:125–40.
3. DeWitt DL, Smith WL. Primary structure of prostaglandin G/H synthase from sheep vesicular gland determined from the complementary DNA sequence. Proc Natl Acad Sci USA. 1988;85:1412–16.
4. Merlie JP, Fagan D, Mudd J, Needleman P. Isolation and characterization of the complementary DNA for sheep seminal vesicle prostaglandin endoperoxide synthase (cyclooxygenase). J Biol Chem. 1988;263:3550–3.
5. Yokoyama C, Takai T, Tanabe T. Primary structure of sheep prostaglandin endoperoxide synthase deduced from cDNA sequences. FEBS Lett. 1988;231:347–51.
6. DeWitt DL, El-Harith EA, Kraemer SA et al. The aspirin and heme-binding sites of ovine and murine prostaglandin endoperoxide synthases. J Biol Chem. 1990;265:5192–8.
7. Yokoyama C, Tanabe T. Cloning of human gene encoding prostaglandin endoperoxide synthase and primary structure of the enzyme. Biochem Biophys Res Commun. 1989;165:888–94.
8. Xie WL, Chipman JG, Robertson DL, Erikson RL, Simmons DL. Expression of a mitogen-responsive gene encoding prostaglandin synthase is regulated by mRNA splicing. Proc Natl Acad Sci USA. 1988;88:2692–6.
9. Kujubu DA, Fletcher BS, Varnum BC, Lim RW, Herschman HR. TIS10, a phorbol ester tumor promoter-inducible mRNA from Swiss 3T3 cells, encodes a novel prostaglandin synthase/cyclooxygenase homologue. J Biol Chem. 1991;266:12866–72.
10. Hla T, Neilson K. Human cyclooxygenase-2 cDNA. Proc Natl Acad Sci USA. 1992;89:7384–8.
11. Vane JR. Inhibition of prostaglandin synthesis as a mechanism of action of aspirin-like drugs. Nature New Biol. 1971;231:232–5.
12. Flower RJ, Vane JR. Inhibition of prostaglandin biosynthesis. Biochem Pharmacol. 1974;23:1439–50.
13. Vane JR, Botting RM. New insights into the mode of action of anti-inflammatory drugs. Inflamm Res. 1995;44:1–10.
14. Futaki N, Takahashi S, Yokoyama M, Arai I, Higuchi S, Otomo S. NS-398, a new anti-inflammatory agent, selectively inhibits prostaglandin G/H synthase/cyclooxygenase (COX-2) activity in vitro. Prostaglandins. 1994;47:55–9.
15. Klein T, Nüsing RM, Pfeilschifter J, Ullrich V. Selective inhibition of cyclooxygenase-2. Biochem Pharmacol. 1994;48:1605–10.
16. Gans KR, Galbraith W, Flower RJ et al. Anti-inflammatory and safety profile of DuP-697, a novel orally effective prostaglandin synthesis inhibitor. J Pharmacol Exp Ther. 1990;254:180–7.
17. Boyce S, Chan C-C, Gordon R et al. L-745,337 – a selective inhibitor of cyclooxygenase-2 elicits antinociception but not gastric-ulceration in rats. Neuropharmacology. 1994;33:1609–11.
18. Chan C-C, Boyce S, Brideau C et al. Pharmacology of a selective cyclooxygenase-2 inhibitor, L-745,337: a novel nonsteroidal anti-inflammatory agent with an ulcerogenic sparing effect in rat and nonhuman primate stomach. J Pharmacol Exp Ther. 1995;274:1531–7.
19. Prasit P, Black WC, Chan C-C et al. L-745,337, a selective cyclooxygenase-2 inhibitor. Med Chem Res. 1995;5:364–74.
20. Leblanc Y, Gauthier J-Y, Ethier D et al. Synthesis and biological evaluation of 2,3-diarylthiophenes as selective COX-2 and COX-1 inhibitors. Bioorg Med Chem Lett. 1995;5:2123–8.
21. Gauthier JY, Leblanc Y, Black C et al. Synthesis and biological evaluation of 2,3-diarylthio-

phenes as selective COX-2. Part II: replacing the heterocycle. Bioorg Med Chem Lett. 1996;6: 87–92.

22. Reitz DB, Huang H-C, Li JJ et al. Selective cyclooxygenase inhibitors: novel 4-spiro 1,2-diarylcyclopentenes are potent and orally active COX-2 inhibitors. Bioorg Med Chem Lett. 1995; 5:8767–872.

23. Seibert K, Zhang Y, Leahy S et al. Pharmacological and biochemical demonstration of the role of cyclooxygenase-2 in inflammation and pain. Proc Natl Acad Sci USA. 1994;91:12013–17.

24. Picott D, Loll PJ, Garavito RM. The x-ray crystal structure of the membrane protein prostaglandin H2 synthase-2. Nature. 1994;367:243–9.

25. Mancini JA, Riendeau D, Falgueyret J-P, Vickers PJ, O'Neill G. Arginine 120 of prostaglandin G/H synthase-1 is required for the inhibition by nonsteroidal anti-inflammatory drugs containing a carboxylic acid moiety. J Biol Chem. 1995;270:29372–7.

26. Ouellet M, Percival DM. Effect of inhibitor time-dependency on selectivity towards cyclo-oxygenase isoforms. Biochem J. 1995;306:247–51.

27. Copeland RA, Williams JM, Giannaras J et al. Mechanism of selective inhibition of the inducible isoform of prostaglandin G/H synthase. Proc Natl Acad Sci USA. 1994;91:11202–6.

28. Fries JF. NSAID gastropathy: the second most deadly rheumatic disease? J Rheumatol. 1991;28(Suppl.):6–10.

29. Sandor Z, Szabo S. Pharmacological approaches and pathogenetic basis of NSAID gastropathy: prevention and treatment. Pract Gastroenterol. 1991;15:30–43.

30. Robert A, Ruwart M. Effects of prostaglandins on the digestive system. In: Lee JB, editor. Prostaglandins. New York: Elsevier North Holland, Inc; 1982:113–76.

31. Fletcher JR. Eicosanoids. Arch Surg. 1993;128:1192–6.

32. Wallace JL. Prostaglandins, NSAIDs, and cytoprotection. Gastroenterol Clin N Am. 1992;21: 631–41.

33. Bennett A. Prostaglandins and the alimentary tract. In: Karim SMM, editor. Prostaglandins: Physiological, Pharmacological and Pathological Aspects. Baltimore: University Park Press; 1976:247–76.

34. Eberhart CE, DuBois RN. Eicosanoids and the gastrointestinal tract. Gastroenterology. 1995; 109:285–301.

35. Kargman SL, O'Neill GP, Vickers PJ, Evans JF, Mancini JA, Jothy S. Expression of prostaglandin G/H synthase-1 and -2 protein in human colon cancer. Cancer Res. 1995;55: 2556–9.

36. Kargman S, Charleson S, Cartwright M et al. Prostaglandin G/H synthase-1 and -2 in rat, dog, monkey and human gastrointestinal tracts: localization, enzymatic activity and inhibition by NSAIDs. Gastroenterology. In press.

37. Eberhart CE, Coffey RJ, Radhika A, Giardiello FM, Ferrenback S, Dubois RN. Up-regulation of cyclooxygenase-2 gene expression in human colorectal adenomas and adenocarcinomas. Gastroenterology. 1994;107:1183–8.

38. Sano H, Kawahito Y, Wilder RI et al. Expression of cyclooxygenase-1 and -2 in human colorectal cancer. Cancer Res. 1995;55:3785–9.

39. Langenbach R, Morham SG, Tiano HF et al. Prostaglandin synthase-1 gene disruption in mice reduces arachidonic acid-induced inflammation and indomethacin-induced gastric ulceration. Cell. 1995;83:483–92.

40. Clive DM, Staff JS. Renal syndromes associated with nonsteroidal anti-inflammatory drugs. N Engl J Med. 1984;310:563–72.

41. Jackson EK, Branch RA, Margolius HS, Oates JA. Physiological functions of the renal prostaglandin, renin and kallikrein systems. In: Seldin DW, Giebisch G, editors. The Kidney, Physiology and Pathophysiology. New York: Raven Press; 1985:613–36.

42. Murray MD, Brater DC. Renal toxicity of the nonsteroidal anti-inflammatory drugs. Annu Rev Pharmacol Toxicol. 1993;33:435–65.

43. Harris RC, McKanna JA, Akai Y, Jacobson HR, Dubois RN. Cyclooxygenase-2 is associated with the macula densa of rat kidney and increased with salt restriction. J Clin Invest. 1994; 94:2504–10.

44. Seibert K, Masferrer JL, Needleman R, Salvemini D. Pharmacological manipulation of cyclo-oxygenase-2 in the inflamed hydronephrotic kidney. Br J Pharmacol. 1996;117:1016–20.

7 Characteristics of cyclooxygenase-1 and cyclooxygenase-2-deficient mice

S. G. MORHAM and R. LANGENBACH

The prostaglandins (PGs) are a diverse group of autocrine and paracrine hormones that mediate many cellular and physiological processes. Prostaglandin H_2 (PGH_2) is an obligate intermediate in formation of prostaglandins[1], the formation of which from arachidonic acid (AA) is catalysed by prostaglandin H synthase, an enzyme with two known isoforms, cyclooxygenase (COX) 1 and COX-2. The genes coding for COX-1 and COX-2 in the mouse are *ptgs1* and *ptgs2*. These enzymes are thought to be the primary enzymatic targets for non-steroid anti-inflammatory drugs (NSAIDs)[2–4]. Since PGH_2 is the major precursor for further PG synthesis, inhibition of cyclooxygenase by NSAIDs leads to a reduction in the production of PGs. Although COX-1 and COX-2 share similar amino acid sequences and enzymatic functions[5–8], their physiological roles are thought to be quite different[9].

COX-1 is constitutively expressed in most tissues[10,11], but at different levels in various cell types. Immunofluorescence data indicate that COX-1 is the isoform expressed in kidney, stomach, vascular smooth muscle[9] and platelets[14]. Enzyme expression usually remains at fairly constant levels, although dramatic changes can occur in certain cells after stimulation with growth factors or other agents[12,13]. COX-2 has a markedly different expression pattern. The enzyme is normally undetectable in most tissues, but it can be expressed at high levels in macrophages and certain other cell types after induction with a variety of substances, including inflammatory mediators and mitogens[15–22].

Current theory suggests that COX-1 inhibition by NSAIDs results in a reduction of PGs which are necessary for cytoprotection of the gastric mucosa and for normal kidney function. This reduction is thought to result in the toxic effects of gastric ulceration and nephrotoxicity associated with long term NSAID use. In addition, the induction of COX-2 by inflammatory mediators and its inhibition by the anti-inflammatory agent dexamethasone has led to the hypothesis that inhibition of COX-2 by NSAIDs is responsible for the anti-inflammatory effects of these drugs. It is interesting to examine these hypotheses in light of the data from COX-1 and COX-2-deficient mice which are unable to synthesize PGs from each of the individual isoforms.

MOLECULAR CHARACTERIZATION OF COX-1 AND COX-2-DEFICIENT ANIMALS

Homologous recombination resulted in the interruption of exon 11 in *ptgs-1*. Germline transmission of this mutation into mice was confirmed by PCR and Southern blotting.

Analysis of transcript levels by Northern blotting demonstrated the absence of COX-1 message from several tissues of homozygous mutant animals. Furthermore, COX-1 protein was not detected by Western blotting with an anti-COX-1-specific antibody. Basal levels of PG synthesis in peritoneal macrophages from COX-1-deficient mice were < 1% of that in wild-type animals[23]. We concluded that the *ptgs1* gene had been completely inactivated in these animals.

An insertion which interrupts the coding sequence in exon 8 of *ptgs2* was introduced into the mouse genome, and its germline transmission was confirmed by PCR and Southern blotting. In addition to the insertion, we introduced a 104 bp deletion in exon 8 that eliminated the nucleotides encoding tyrosine-371 and histidine-374[33]. These amino acids are both crucial for cyclooxygenase activity[24,25]. Neither COX-2 transcript nor protein could be detected by Northern blotting or Western blotting in COX-2-deficient peritoneal macrophages. While higher levels of PGs could be readily induced by lipopolysaccharide (LPS) in wild-type peritoneal macrophages, the cells from COX-2-deficient animals showed only basal levels of synthesis after LPS stimulation. We concluded that this mutation completely inactivates *ptgs2* in these mice.

EFFECTS OF COX-1 AND COX-2 DEFICIENCY ON THE GASTROINTESTINAL TRACT

Prostaglandins have long been thought to be necessary for maintenance of the stomach mucosa and for proper gastric function[26]. Current theory suggests that gastric ulceration caused by NSAIDs is due to their inhibition of COX-1-derived PG synthesis[27–29]. A corollary of this hypothesis is that elimination of the COX-1 PG synthesis pathway should result in spontaneous gastric ulceration. However, examination of over 20 COX-1-deficient animals revealed no pathology in the stomach, small intestine or large intestine. Examination of these same organs for inflammatory histopathology showed no evidence of inflammation. COX-1-deficient mice had a pH of 1.0–2.5, compared with 2.5–3.5 in wild-type mice, showing that a reduction in stomach acidity is not responsible for the lack of ulceration found in COX-1-deficient animals.

To determine whether a compensatory mechanism had restored COX activity in the absence of COX-1, the possibility of COX-2 up-regulation in COX-1-deficient animals was investigated; no such up-regulation was observed[23]. Levels of PGE_2 and 6-ketoPGF$_{1\alpha}$ (a breakdown product used for measurement of prostacyclin) in the stomachs of COX-1-deficient mice were < 1% of that found in wild-type animals. PG levels < 1% of normal were also found in wild-type mice which received the NSAID indomethacin. Thus, levels of PGs in the stomachs of COX-1-deficient animals and in wild-type animals treated with indomethacin were similar, yet the NSAID-treated wild-type mice had a much higher incidence of ulceration than the COX-1-deficient mice[23]. Surprisingly, COX-1-deficient mice were more resistant to acute indomethacin-induced gastric ulceration than were wild-type mice[23]. The absence of spontaneous ulceration in mice lacking the basal levels of PGs produced by COX-1 demonstrates that PGs are not required for gastric cytoprotection. This renders unlikely the hypothesis that gastritis associated with NSAIDs is induced by inhibition of COX-1-derived PG synthesis.

Histological examination of 20 COX-2-deficient animals also showed no evidence of pathology on the mucosal surfaces of the stomach, small intestine or large intestine. These data indicate that the relationship between NSAID-induced ulceration and COX activity is complex, and that the inhibition of cyclooxygenase by NSAIDs is not equivalent to the elimination of PG synthesis by either *ptgs1* or *ptgs2* inactivation in this instance.

Several possibilities exist which can explain the data obtained from these mice. Altered regulation of inducible nitric oxide synthase, various cytokines or unknown factors could account for the lack of ulceration in COX-1-deficient mice. The possibility also exists that inhibition of both COX enzymes is necessary for gastric ulceration. Alternatively, it is possible that the interaction of the NSAID with the COX enzyme causes ulceration by forming a drug–enzyme complex which inhibits another pathway or leads to the production of an aberrant product (or products). Whatever the cause of indomethacin-induced gastritis, it is clear that the ulceration proceeds by mechanisms in addition to, or other than, inhibition of COX-1.

INFLAMMATORY RESPONSES IN COX-1- OR COX-2-DEFICIENT MICE

COX-1 is considered to perform primarily housekeeping functions, while COX-2 is the isoform associated with inflammation[27–30]. Mice deficient in either COX-1 or COX-2 provide models for determining the relative contributions of the two isoforms to the inflammatory process. When arachidonic acid (AA) was administered topically to the inner side of the ear COX-1-deficient mice showed only 30% of the inflammatory response found in wild-type mice[31,32]. This response was maximal by 2 h and declined to basal levels by 5 h after AA administration. These findings implicate COX-1 in AA-induced inflammation. AA can be immediately metabolized by the constitutively expressed COX-1 isoform to PGH_2 and further metabolized to PGE_2, which would then be expected to cause oedema and neutrophil invasion. Since COX-1 is not expressed in the mutant mice, there is an attenuation of this inflammatory response. These data demonstrate a role for COX-1 in the inflammatory process, although it is not yet clear under which circumstances this role is important.

COX-2-deficient mice do not have an altered AA-induced inflammatory response when compared with wild-type mice. The maximal inflammatory response occurs at 2 h; this is likely to be before the expression of COX-2. The decline of the response over a 5 h period would coincide with the possible induction of COX-2, making it unlikely that COX-2 plays a role in topically induced inflammation.

Neither COX-deficient mouse model shows an altered inflammatory response to topical treatment with tetradecanoyl phorbol acetate (TPA), which is maximal at 6 h and declines over 24 h to basal levels. TPA is known to induce COX-2 expression and for this reason it is somewhat surprising that homozygous COX-2 deficiency had no effect on the inflammatory response. However, it is possible that TPA induces phospholipases which liberate AA for metabolism by either COX isoform. These data indicate that either both isoforms can complement the absence of the other to contribute to TPA-induced inflammation, or that neither enzyme is required for this process.

A spontaneous peritonitis was found in seven of 20 COX-2-deficient mice examined[33], but in none of 40 wild-type mice. This may indicate that the COX-2-deficient genotype combined with another factor, possibly environmental in nature, leads to this bacterial peritonitis. Histological examination revealed classical signs of inflammation in response to invasion of the peritoneal cavity by bacteria, with regions of oedema, infiltration of neutrophils into interstitial spaces and serosal exudation in the superficial tissues of the viscera and in the retroperitoneum. These conditions would be expected in a normal inflammatory response to bacterial infection. While clearly the presence of COX-2 is not required for these inflammatory responses, the enzyme may be necessary for the prevention or amelioration of this condition. It has been suggested that the enhanced release of eicosanoids by infiltrating cells modulates interactions between mononuclear cells, fibroblasts, platelets and lymphocytes. These interactions may then result in the release of inflammatory mediators coupled to arachidonate metabolism that collectively influence tissue injury[34]. Aberrant modulation of the eicosanoids as a result of COX-2 deficiency could alter cell–cell interactions, resulting in peritonitis. We do not at present understand the nature of this spontaneous peritonitis; however, we are now examining the mice to investigate the possibility that they are immunocompromised in some manner.

Dinchuk et al. have demonstrated that the inflammatory response to carrageenan-induced paw oedema in COX-2-deficient mice is similar to that of wild-type mice[35]. These authors concluded that this experimentally induced inflammation was COX-2 independent. Thus, several experimental models of inflammation fail to show any difference between COX-2-deficient and wild-type mice, and COX-2-deficient mice show classic inflammatory responses to the invasion of the peritoneum by bacteria.

The data from COX-1-deficient animals show a decrease in inflammation following topical administration of AA but not TPA. COX-2-deficient animals show no differences in inflammation compared to wild-type using the models thus far evaluated. This indicates that the circumstances of tissue injury are likely to influence which isoform acts in an accompanying inflammatory response.

KIDNEY PATHOLOGY IN COX-2-DEFICIENT MICE

The kidneys of COX-2 homozygous mutant mice were small, pale and had a granular appearance on the capsular surface. All showed lesions of mild to marked severity, except those from mice that were only 3 days old. In its mildest form, the nephropathy was characterized by multifocal areas of abnormal subcapsular parenchyma comprising small immature glomeruli and tubules, consistent with nephron hypoplasia. In some cases, the cortex appeared thinned and the number of glomeruli was reduced in comparison to wild-type kidneys. Glomeruli not within the hypoplastic zone were frequently enlarged. Other pathological findings included cortical areas of tubular atrophy and regeneration, protein and cellular casts within tubular lumens, tubular dilation, interstitial inflammation and fibrosis and papillary mineralization. In general, these changes were more severe in males than in females and increased in severity with increasing age. Kidneys from 8-week-old COX-2-deficient animals had a few small scattered foci of tubular atrophy and interstitial fibrosis; these were not present in 6-week-old COX-2-deficient mice. The single homozygous mutant male which survived to necropsy at 16 weeks of age had severe focal interstitial fibrosis and tubular atrophy associated with focal segmental and global glomerular sclerosis. The renal histology of 3-day-old COX-2-deficient mice did not differ from that of wild-type mice; in particular, these mice had a normal subcapsular zone of immature nephrogenic tissue. In contrast, mice aged 6 weeks or more showed abnormal nephron hypoplasia in the subcapsular region. Thus, kidneys of the COX-2-deficient mice show progressive deterioration and developmental abnormality with increasing age.

We have established that 3-day-old COX-2-deficient mice do not show the kidney pathology found in older animals: kidney development continues for several weeks after birth, however. The observation of renal abnormalities in COX-2-deficient animals of at least 6 weeks of age suggests a postnatal maturation arrest in the subcapsular nephrogenic zone that would normally continue to generate nephrons up to 4 weeks postnatally. Such an arrest would result in a subcapsular zone of hypoplastic glomeruli, and appears to cause compensatory hypertrophy of those glomeruli and tubules that developed prior to the maturation arrest. The glomerular sclerosis and associated tubulointerstitial injury observed in the 16-week-old homozygous mutant may have resulted from a work overload on the reduced number of functional nephrons.

Thus, a possible explanation for these findings is that total absence of COX-2 impairs postnatal differentiation of the kidneys within the subcapsular nephrogenic zone. The reduced number of nephrons means that those nephrons that are present have an increased workload. This leads first to hypertrophy and eventually to glomerular sclerosis[36]. This type of glomerular compensatory hypertrophy and subsequent sclerosis occurs following experimental reduction in the number of nephrons in utero[37] or after birth[36]. It is most severe when the reduction in nephrons occurs early[38]. We are currently investigating the role of COX-2 and PG synthesis in kidney development.

FERTILITY IN COX-1- AND COX-2-DEFICIENT ANIMALS

Prostaglandins have important functions in various stages of the reproductive process, including ovulation, spermatogenesis and parturition[39–41]. Which isoform is involved in these processes is only partially clear at the present time; however these mice offer an excellent model in which to investigate the relative importance of the two isoforms in the reproductive process.

Male COX-1- or COX-2-deficient mice can both effectively impregnate wild-type or heterozygous mutant females, so the role of these isoforms in spermatogenesis is not essential. The fertility of COX-1-deficient females is not affected except when two homozygous mutants are mated. This mating produced a 90% decrease in pup survival and showed an increased length of labour, which may be responsible for the pup mortality. No obvious pathology was found in the pups which died and surviving mice were developmentally normal. Heterozygous male by homozygous female matings resulted in normal litter sizes and pup survival. This indicates that the presence of prostaglandins from 50% of the COX 1 heterozygous offspring can complement the deficiency of the mother, resulting in normal labour and parturition.

COX-2-deficient females are infertile, and this seems to be due to a lack of ovulation. Female infertility has also been found in other COX-2-deficient animals[35].

CONCLUSIONS

COX-1- and COX-2-deficient mice provide model systems for a variety of scientific investigations, including studies of inflammation, NSAIDs, development and fertility. The data from these animal models are difficult to reconcile with the notion of COX-1 regulating housekeeping functions, such as gastric cytoprotection and normal renal maintenance, while COX-2 regulates inflammation. It is likely that both COX isoforms have a role in the inflammatory process, each under particular circumstances of tissue injury. It is unlikely that the gastric side effects of NSAIDs are caused by inhibition of PG synthesis alone. The roles of the individual COX isoforms in cellular and physiological biology are more complex than previously surmised, and there is a need to reassess current theory on the functions of COX-1 and COX-2.

The differences between mouse and human biology pertaining to the roles of the COX isoforms and PG synthesis are a caveat which must be taken into account when assessing these mutant models. However, studies of COX-1- and COX-2-deficient mice can indicate future directions for scientific inquiry. The data thus derived from these animals should be of great value for elucidating the functions of the two COX isoforms and also to research directed at the development of improved NSAIDs.

Acknowledgements

S.G.M. is an American Cancer Society Fellow (#PF-3973) in the laboratory of Dr Oliver Smithies, Excellence Professor of Pathology at the University of North Carolina at Chapel Hill. Work on COX-1- and COX-2-deficient mice was supported by grants GM20069 and HL49227 from the NIH to O. Smithies. We also wish to thank C. Loftin, H. Tiano and P. Chulada for communicating unpublished data.

References

1. Smith WL. The eicosanoids and their biochemical mechanisms of action. Biochem J. 1989;259: 315–24.
2. Flower RJ, Vane JR. Inhibition of prostaglandin synthetase in brain explains the antipyretic activity of paracetamol (4-acetamidophenol). Nature. 1972;240:410–11.
3. Flower R, Gryglewski R, Herbaczynska-Cedro K, Vane JR. Effects of anti-inflammatory drugs on prostaglandin biosynthesis. Nature. 1972;238:104–6.
4. Dewitt DL, Meade FA, Smith WL. PGH synthase isozyme selectivity: the potential safer non-steroidal antiinflammatory drugs. Am J Med. 1993;95:40s–4s.
5. O'Banion MK, Winn VD, Young DA. cDNA cloning and functional activity of a glucocorticoid-regulated inflammatory cyclooxygenase. Proc Natl Acad Sci USA. 1992;89:4888–92.
6. Ryseck RP, Raynoscheck C, Macdonald-Bravo H, Dorfman K, Mattei MG, Bravo R. Identification of an immediate early gene, pghs-B, whose protein product has prostaglandin synthase/cyclooxygenase activity. Cell Growth Diff. 1992;3:443–50.
7. Fletcher BS, Kujubu DA, Perrin DM, Herschman HR. Structure of the mitogen-inducible TIS10 gene and demonstration that the TIS10-encoded protein is a functional prostaglandin G/H synthase. J Biol Chem. 1992;267:4338–44.

8. Hsi LC, Hoganson CW, Babcock GT, Smith WL. Characterization of a tyrosyl radical in prostaglandin endoperoxide synthase-2. Biochem Biophys Res Commun. 1994;202:1592–8.
9. Smith WL, Meade EA, DeWitt DL. Interactions of PGH synthase isozymes -1 and -2 with NSAIDs. Ann NY Acad Sci. 1994;744:50–7.
10. Simmons DL, Xie W, Chipman JG, Evett GE. Multiple cyclooxygenase cloning of a mitogen-inducible form. In: JM Bailey, editor. Prostaglandins, Leukotrienes, Lipoxins and PAF. New York: Plenum Press. 1991:67–78.
11. O'Neill PO, Ford-Hutchinson AW. Expression of mRNA for cyclooxygenase-1 and cyclo-oxygenase-2 in human tissues. FEBS Lett. 1993;330:156–60.
12. DeWitt DL. Prostaglandin endoperoxide synthase: regulation of enzyme expression. Biochim Biophys Acta. 1991;1083:121–34.
13. Smith CJ, Morrow JD, Roberts LJ, Marnett LJ. Differentiation of monocytoid THP-1 cells with phorbol ester induces expression of prostaglandin endoperoxide synthase-1 (COX-1). Biochem Biophys Res Commun. 1993;192:787–93.
14. Funk CD, Funk LB, Kennedy ME, Pong AS, Fitzgerald GA. Human platelet/erythroleukemia cell prostaglandin G/H synthase: cDNA cloning, expression and gene chromosomal assignment. FASEB J. 1991;5:2304–12.
15. Lee SH, Soyoola E, Chanmugam P et al. Selective expression of a mitogen-inducible cyclo-oxygenase in macrophages stimulated with lipopolysaccharide. J Biol Chem. 1992;267:25934–8.
16. Fu JY, Masferrer JL, Seibert K, Raz A, Needleman P. The induction and suppression of prosta-glandin H2 synthase (cyclooxygenase) in human monocytes. J Biol Chem. 1990;265:16737–40.
17. Evett GE, Xie W, Chipman JG, Robertson DL, Simmons DL. Prostaglandin G/H synthase isoenzyme 2 expression in fibroblasts: regulation by dexamethasone, mitogens and oncogenes. Arch Biochem Biophys. 1993;306:169–77.
18. Kujubu DA, Fletcher BS, Varnum BC, Lim RW, Hershman HR. TIS10, a phorbol ester tumor promoter-inducible mRNA from Swiss 3T3 cells, encodes a novel prostaglandin synthase/cyclo-oxygenase homologue. J Biol Chem. 1991;266:12866–72.
19. Masferrer JL, Siebert K, Zweifel B, Needleman P. Endogenous glucocorticoids regulate an inducible cyclooxygenase enzyme. Proc Natl Acad Sci USA. 1992;89:3917–21.
20. Sano H, Hla T, Maier JAM et al. In vivo cyclooxygenase expression in synovial tissues of patients with rheumatoid arthritis and osteoarthritis and rats with adjuvant and streptococcal cell wall arthritis. J Clin Invest. 1992;89:97–108.
21. O'Sullivan GM, Huggins FM, Meade FA, DeWitt DL, McCall CE. Lipopolysaccharide priming of alveolar macrophages for enhanced synthesis of prostanoids involves induction of a novel prostaglandin H synthase. Biochem Biophys Res Commun. 1992;187:1123–7.
22. O'Sullivan GM, Chilton FH, Huggins EM, McCall CE. Lipopolysaccharide induces prostaglandin II synthase-2 in alveolar macrophages. J Biol Chem. 1992;267:14547–50.
23. Langenbach R, Morham SG, Tiano HF et al. Prostaglandin synthase 1 gene disruption in mice reduces arachidonic acid induced inflammation and indomethacin induced gastric ulceration. Cell. 1995;83:483–92.
24. Shimokawa T, Kulmacz RJ, DeWitt DL, Smith WL. Tyrosine 385 of prostaglandin endoperoxide synthase is required for cyclooxygenase catalysis. J Biol Chem. 1990;265:20073–6.
25. Shimokawa T, Smith WL. Essential histidines of prostaglandin endoperoxide synthase. J Biol Chem. 1990;265:6168–73.
26. Robert A. An intestinal disease produced experimentally by a prostaglandin deficiency. Gastro-enterology. 1975;69:1045–7.
27. Masferrer JL, Zweifel BS, Manning PT et al. Selective inhibition of inducible cyclooxygenase 2 in vivo is antiinflammatory and nonulcerogenic. Proc Natl Acad Sci USA. 1994;91:3228–32.
28. Vane J. Towards a better aspirin. Nature. 1994;367:215–16.
29. Seibert K, Zhang Y, Leahy K et al. Pharmacological and biochemical demonstration of the role of cyclooxygenase 2 in inflammation and pain. Proc Natl Acad Sci USA. 1994;91:12013–17.
30. DeWitt DL, Smith WL. Cloning of sheep and mouse prostaglandin endoperoxide synthases. Methods Enzymol. 1990;187:469–79.
31. Gad SC, Dunn BJ, Dobbs DW, Reilly C, Walsh RW. Development and validation of an alterna-tive dermal sensitization test: the mouse ear swelling test (MEST). Toxicol Appl Pharmacol. 1986;84:93–114.
32. Opas EE, Bonney RJ, Humes JL. Prostaglandin and leukotriene synthesis in mouse ears inflamed

by arachidonic acid. J Invest Dermatol. 1985;84:253–6.

33. Morham SG, Langenbach R, Loftin CD et al. Prostaglandin synthase 2 gene disruption causes severe renal pathology in the mouse. Cell. 1995;83:473–82.

34. Seibert K, Masferrer JL, Jiya F, Honda A, Raz A, Needleman P. The biochemical and pharmacological manipulation of cellular cyclooxygenase (COX) activity. Adv Prostaglandin, Thromboxane Leukotriene Res. 1991;21A:45–51.

35. Dinchuk JE, Car BD, Focht RJ et al. Renal abnormalities and an altered inflammatory response in mice lacking cyclooxygenase II. Nature. 1995;378:406–9.

36. Brenner BM. Nephron adaptation to renal injury or ablation. Am J Physiol. 1985;249:F324–37.

37. Gilbert T, Lelievre-Pegorier M, Merlet-Benichou C. Long-term effects of mild oligonephronia induced in utero by gentamicin in the rat. Pediatr Res. 1991;30:450–6.

38. Celsi G, Jakobsson B, Aperia A. Influence of age on compensatory renal growth in rats. Pediatr Res. 1986;20:347–50.

39. Thorburn GD. The placenta, prostaglandins and parturition: A review. Reprod Fert Dev. 1991;3:227–94.

40. Sirois J, Simmons DL, Richards JS. Hormonal regulation of messenger ribonucleic acid encoding a novel isoform of prostaglandin endoperoxide II synthase in rat preovulatory follicles. J Biol Chem. 1992;267:11586–92.

41. Zahradnik HP, Schafer W, Neulen J et al. The role of eicosanoids in reproduction. Eicosanoids. 1992;5:S56–9.

Figure 1   Crystal of human COX-2 protein. The COX-2 protein from the baculovirus expression system [7] was purified and crystallized as described [5]. The dimensions of the crystal are approximately 0.15×0.10×0.5 mm

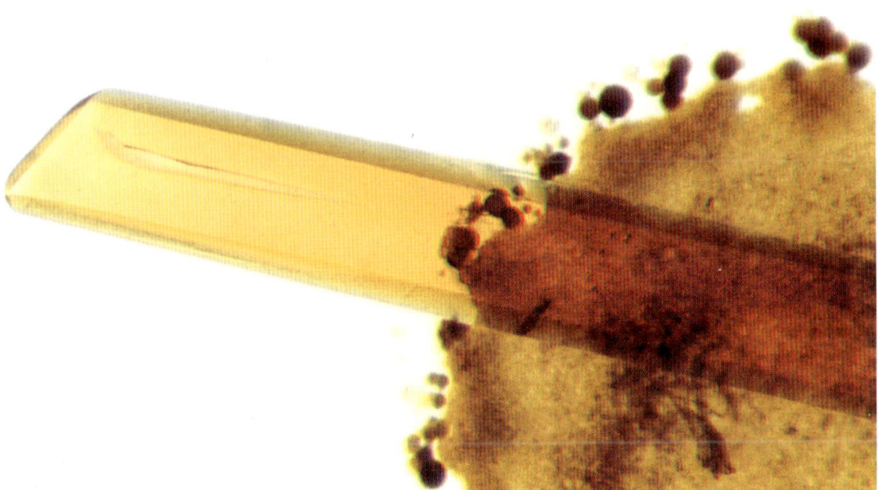

Figure 2   The structure of the human COX-2 dimer shown in a ribbon representation. In each monomer the EGF domain (N-terminal) is coloured yellow, the membrane binding domain is blue and the catalytic domain (C-terminal) is magenta. The haem co-factor, required for peroxidase activity, is shown in CPK representation, coloured orange. The COX-2 inhibitor (green, compound 1) is bound at the NSAID (cyclooxygenase) site. The plane of the lipid membrane is horizontal near the bottom of the diagram and the dimer interface is perpendicular to the plane of the membrane. A rotation of 90° back into the page would provide a view into the NSAID binding site from the membrane

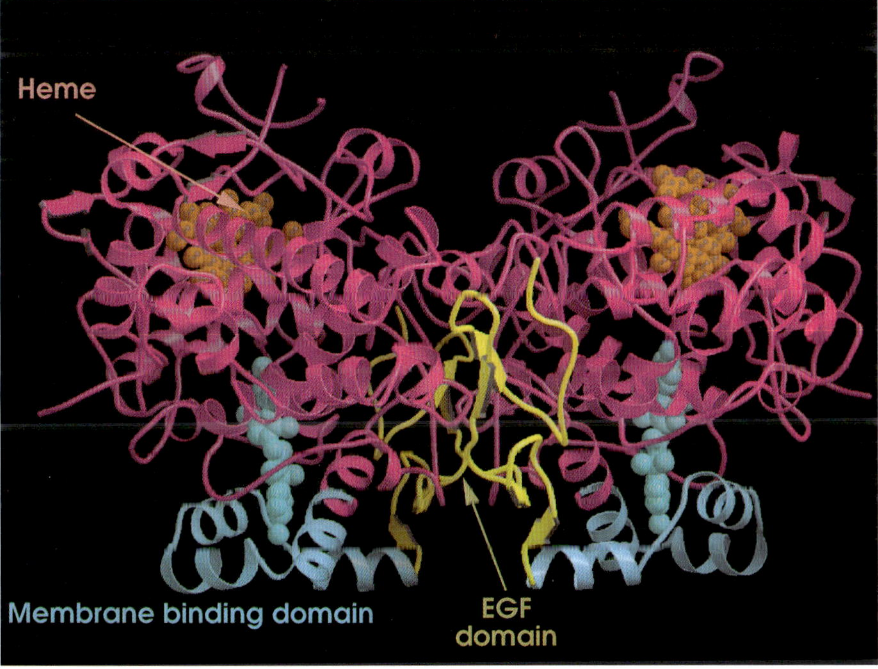

Figure 3   Comparison of the structure and amino acid sequence of human COX-2 and sheep COX-1. (a) The α-carbon ribbon diagram of the human COX-2 (blue) and sheep COX-1 (green) structures are shown superimposed to indicate the overall similarity between the two structures; 0.9 Å root mean square (RMS) deviation for all backbone atoms. (b) Schematic diagram of the domain structure of cyclooxygenase showing the amino acid sequence of sheep COX-1 and human COX-2, the amount of identity between the amino acid sequence and the RMS deviation (all backbone atoms) for the three domains in the X-ray crystal structures

Figure 3(a)

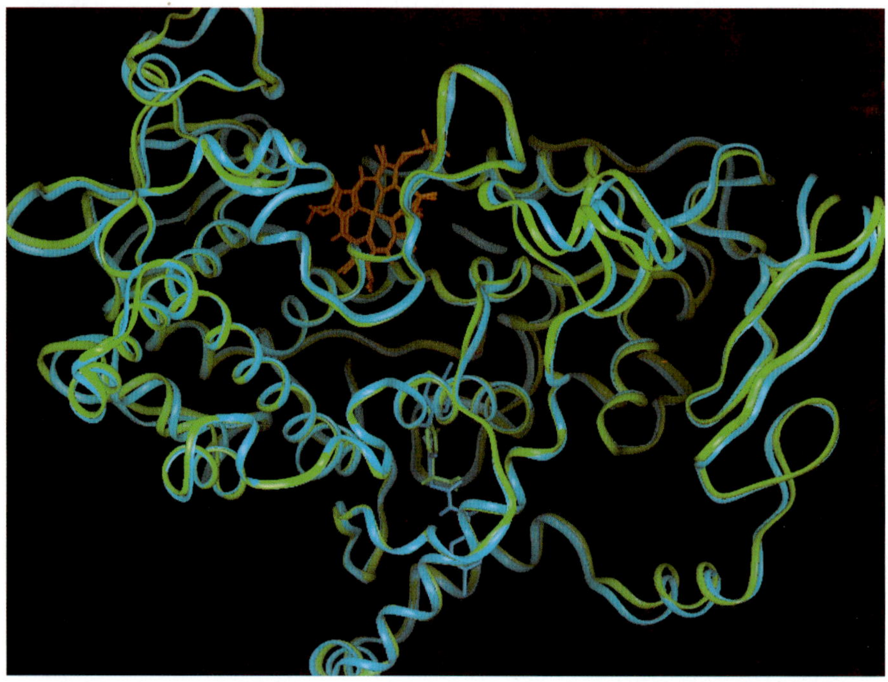

Figure 3(b)

	SIGNAL	EGF	MEMBRANE	CATALYTIC
sheep COX-1	1–24	33–73	74–115	116–585
human COX-2	1–17	18–58	59–101	102–571
% A.A. Identity		59	33	67
RMS deviation (Å)		0.8	0.7	0.9

Figure 4   Close-up view of the NSAID binding site of COX-2. The structures of COX-2[5] and COX-1[16] have been superimposed to show the similarity of the NSAID binding site. Only the ribbon diagram for COX-2 is shown. Amino acid residues that define the NSAID binding site are white for COX-2 and green for COX-1. The amino acids that are different between COX-2 and COX-1 are labelled in yellow; the three letter code is used in labelling the amino acid residues. The dotted white surface indicates the size and shape of the NSAID binding site in the closed COX-2 structure. The dotted green surface is the representation of the NSAID binding site in COX-1[6]

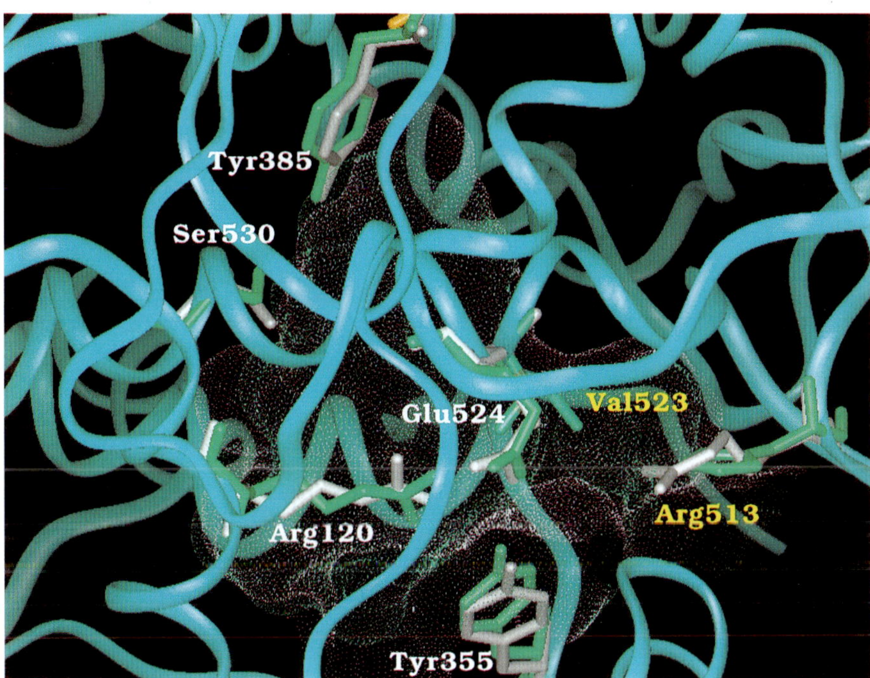

Figure 5(a)   legend overleaf

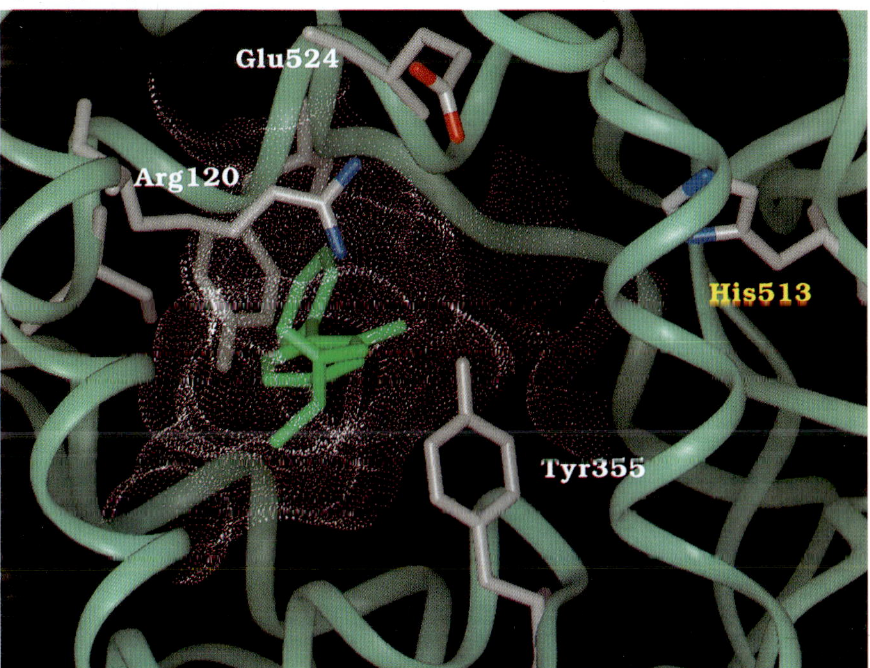

Figure 5 The NSAID binding sites for COX-2 and COX-1. The view of the NSAID binding site is from the bottom, looking up from the membrane binding domain. The dotted surface indicates the NSAID binding site in all structures. The closed conformation of the NSAID binding site in COX-1 (a) and COX-2 (b) and the open (c) conformation of the COX-2 NSAID binding site are shown

Figure 5(b)

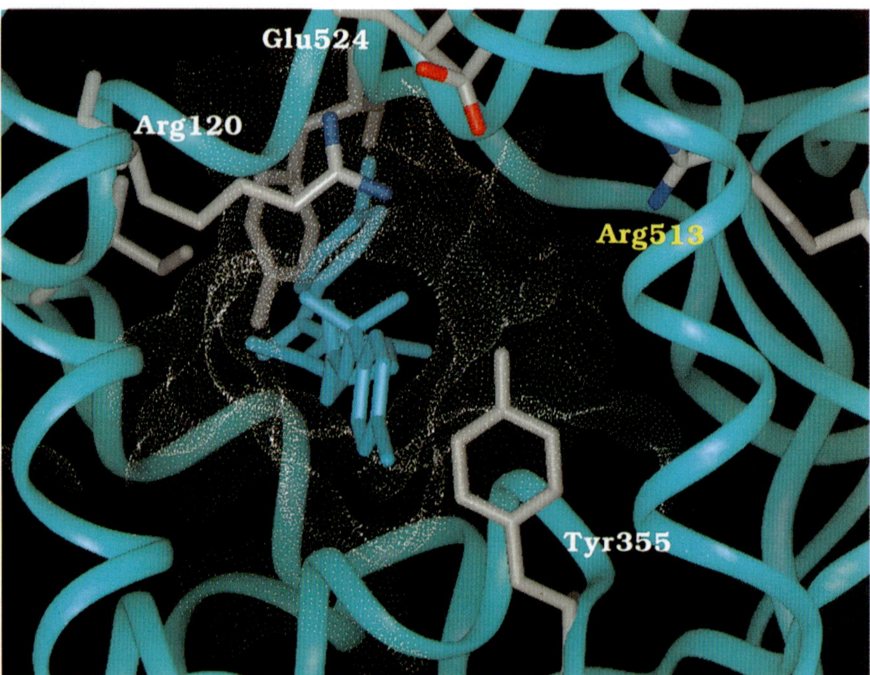

Figure 5(c)

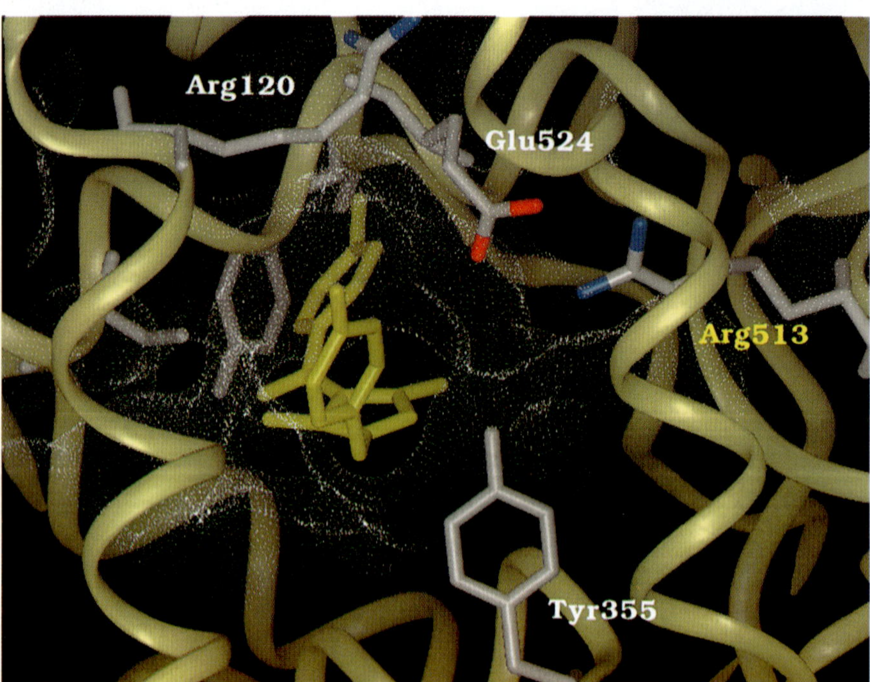

8 X-ray crystal structure of human cyclooxygenase-2

M. F. BROWNER

Non-steroid anti-inflammatory drugs (NSAIDs) exert their beneficial anti-inflammatory actions, as well as their undesirable gastro-intestinal effects, through inhibition of the enzyme prostaglandin H synthase[1], also referred to as cyclooxygenase (COX). The discovery of an inducible COX enzyme (COX-2), distinct from the constitutively expressed enzyme (COX-1)[2,3], has led to the suggestion that a new generation of safer NSAIDs may be developed in the near future. Classical NSAIDs, such as aspirin, flurbiprofen and naproxen, inhibit both COX-1 and COX-2 and are therefore non-selective inhibitors. Simply stated, the COX-2 hypothesis suggests that inhibitors selective for COX-2 over COX-1 should be relatively safer therapeutic agents than currently available NSAIDs. In vivo experiments with selective COX-2 inhibitors support the suggestion that such compounds will have an anti-inflammatory effect without severe gastrointestinal toxicity[4].

The benefits of obtaining structural information at the atomic level for a drug target is now well appreciated: these include the ability to document and exploit differences between closely related enzymes for the design of new inhibitors. In an effort to utilize a structure-based approach in the discovery of selective COX-2 inhibitors, we determined the X-ray crystal structure of human COX-2[5]. Since the crystal structure of sheep COX-1 is known[6], and provided the first atomic details of the cyclooxygenase enzyme, the basis for such an approach in the development of selective COX-2 inhibitors is at hand.

Obtaining atomic resolution structure data for the cyclooxygenase enzymes is made difficult by several properties of these proteins. Cyclooxygenase is a membrane bound homodimeric protein whose monomer has a molecular weight of 72 kDa. The human COX-2 protein obtained from the baculovirus expression system has been shown to be glycosylated and the glycosylation is not homogeneous[7]. Purified human COX-2 protein from the baculovirus system was used in crystallization trials in the absence and presence of various inhibitors. Crystals were obtained under a variety of conditions similar to those reported previously for sheep COX-1[8]. Crystals suitable for X-ray diffraction experiments (Figure 1) were obtained by replacing the non-ionic detergent β-octyl glucoside with octyl pentaoxyethylene[5]. As reported previously for the sheep COX-1 crystals, the human COX-2 crystals are very radiation sensitive at room temperature, making it difficult to collect a complete X-ray diffraction data set with adequate atomic resolution. A procedure for collecting the X-ray diffraction data at low temperatures ($-168°C$) was developed, allowing data at a resolution of more than 3.0 Å to be obtained routinely. The X-ray crystal structure of human COX-2 was

solved by molecular replacement using the sheep COX-1 structure as the starting model[6].

The X-ray structure of human COX-2 is similar to that of sheep COX-1 structure[a]. The cyclooxygenase homodimer is represented in both the COX-1 and COX-2 crystal structures. Figure 2 shows that the COX-2 dimer is oriented such that the plane of the lipid membrane is horizontal and at the bottom, and the dimer interface is perpendicular to the plane of the membrane.

The cyclooxygenase monomer has three distinct domains. The N-terminal domain is a β-sheet domain referred to as the EGF domain because of its similarity to other epidermal growth factor-like protein structures. The next domain contains four helices that are proposed to bind the protein to the lipid membrane[6] and provide access for substrates and inhibitors to the cyclooxygenase active site from within the membrane[5,6]. The third and largest domain is the C-terminal, catalytic domain. The catalytic domain includes both the cyclooxygenase active site, which is also the binding site for NSAIDs[10,11], and the peroxidase active site containing the haem co-factor.

Although the COX-1 and COX-2 proteins are encoded by two different genes[12], the amino acid sequences are closely related (Figure 3). The amino acid sequences of human COX-1 and human COX-2 are 63% identical (78% similar). The human COX-2 and sheep COX-1 amino acid sequences are 62% identical. Given the high degree of amino acid conservation between the COX-1 and COX-2 enzymes, it is not surprising that the structures of human COX-2 and sheep COX-1 are very similar (Figure 3a). The amino acid sequence identity of the catalytic domain of human COX-2 and sheep COX-1 is 67% and the structural details of this domain are also very similar. The structure of the membrane binding domain is also conserved between the two isoenzymes, although the sequence identity is significantly less: there is 33% amino acid identity between the membrane binding helices of human COX-2 and sheep COX-1 (Figure 3b). There is also a single amino acid insertion in the membrane binding domain of COX-2 compared with the COX-1 sequence, which creates a slighly larger loop between the third and fourth helices.

The COX-1 structure revealed an internal channel extending from the centre of the catalytic domain, just below the haem binding site, to the outer surface of the membrane binding helices (Figure 4). This is both the cyclooxygenase binding site and the site where a wide variety of NSAIDs have been shown to bind[5,10,11]. The only amino acid residue lining the NSAID binding site that is not identical between COX-1 and COX-2 is amino acid residue 523, which is an isoleucine (Ile) in COX-1 and valine (Val) in COX-2. This single amino acid substitution has a significant effect on the overall size and shape of the NSAID binding site in COX-2 (Figure 4). Indeed, this single amino acid difference may very well explain the biochemical differences observed between COX-1 and COX-2[13-15].

Structural studies show that selective COX-2 inhibitors are also bound at the NSAID binding site. The positions of the amino acid residues surrounding the

---

[a] The numbering used for the amino acid residues in the COX-2 structure[5] is the same as used for COX-1, Protein Data Bank entry 1PRH[9], the only number difference is the insertion at position 106, which is referred to as 106a.

NSAID binding site of COX-2 are very similar to COX-1 (Figure 4). In particular, amino acid residues arginine (Arg) 120 and tyrosine (Tyr) 355, at the bottom of the NSAID binding site, interact with polar atoms of the inhibitor, in an analogous manner to the interactions with the acid of an NSAID[6,10,11] (Figure 5). This conformation of the NSAID binding site is referred to as the closed conformation in both COX-1[10] (Figure 5a) and in COX-2 (Figure 5b)[5].

A second COX-2 structure, studied using a different selective inhibitor, reveals that an open conformation at the bottom of the NSAID binding site is also possible (Figure 5c). In this structure Arg120 does not participate in the hydrogen bond network that defines the bottom of the NSAID binding site. Apart from the changes at the bottom of the channel, the closed and open COX-2 structures are very similar. Indeed, the overall similarity in the two COX-2 structures suggest that there is structural flexibility between the membrane binding domain and the catalytic domain of cyclooxygenase that can accommodate both open and closed conformations at the bottom of the NSAID binding site.

It has been proposed that both inhibitors and substrate access the NSAID binding site of cyclooxygenase through the membrane. For this to be possible there are probably different conformations of the protein which allow the entrance of rather bulky inhibitors and substrates into a relatively narrow channel. The COX-2 structures provide the first experimental evidence that different conformations of the enzyme can exist. The importance of understanding that a protein can adopt different conformations in response to bound inhibitors should not be underestimated. This type of information will be very valuable in order for a structure-based approach to be successful in developing very selective COX-2 inhibitors.

ACKNOWLEDGMENTS

I thank M. Garavito and P. Loll for advice on the crystallization of human COX-2 and I thank all members of the COX-2 project team, in particular C. Luong and A. Miller in the Molecular Structure Department.

References

1. Vane JR. Inhibition of prostaglandin synthesis as a mechanism of action for aspirin-like drugs. Nature New Biol. 1971;231:232–5.
2. Hla T, Neilson K. Human cyclooxygenase-2 cDNA. Proc Natl Acad Sci. USA. 1992;89:7384–8.
3. Kujubu DA, Fletcher BS, Varnum BC, Lim RW, Herschman HR. TIS10, a phorbol ester tumor promoter-inducible mRNA from swiss 3T3 cells, encodes a novel prostaglandin synthase/ cyclooxygenase. J Biol Chem. 1991;266:12866–72.
4. Masferrer JL, Zweifel BS, Manning PT, et al. Selective inhibition of inducible cyclooxygenase 2 in vivo is antiinflammatory and nonulcerogenic. Proc Natl Acad Sci USA. 1994;91:3228–32.
5. Luong C, Miller A, Barnett J, Chow J, Ramesha C, Browner MF. Flexibility of the NSAID binding site in the structure of human cyclooxygenase-2. Nature Struct Biol. 1996; (in press).
6. Picot D, Loll PJ, Garavito RM. The X-ray crystal structure of the membrane protein prostaglandin H2 synthase-1. Nature. 1994;367:243–9.
7. Barnett J, Chow J, Ives D, et al. Purification, characterization and selective inhibition of human prostaglandin G/H synthase 1 and 2 expressed in the baculovirus system. Biochem Biophys Acta. 1994;1209:130–9.

8. Garavito RM. Crystallizing membrane proteins: Experiments on different systems. In: Michel H, ed. Crystallization of Membrane Proteins. CRC Press, Boca Raton. 1991:89–105.
9. Abola EE, Berstein FC, Bryant SH, Koetzle TF, Weng J. Protein Data Bank. In: Allen FH, Bergerhoff G, Sievers R, ed. Crystallographic Databases – Information Content, Software Systems, Scientific Applications. Bonn: Data Commission of the International Union of Crystallography, 1987:107–32.
10. Loll PJ, Picot D, Ekabo O, Garavito RM. Synthesis and use of iodinated nonsteroidal anti-inflammatory drug analogs as crystallographic probes of the prostaglandin H2 cyclooxygenase active site. Biochemistry. 1996;35:7330–40.
11. Loll PJ, Picot D, Garavito RM. The structural basis of aspirin activity inferred from the crystal structure of inactivated prostaglandin H_2 synthase. Nature Struct Biol. 1995;2:637–42.
12. Tazawa R, Xu XM, Wu KK, Wang LH. Characterization of the genomic structure, chromosomal location and promoter of human prostaglandin H synthase-2 gene. Biochem Biophys Res Commun. 1994;203:190–9.
13. Mancini JA, O'Neill GP, Bayly C, Vickers PJ. Mutation of serine-516 in human prostaglandin G/H synthase-2 to methionine and aspirin acetylation of this residue stimulates 15-R-HETE synthesis. FEBS Lett. 1994;342:33–7.
14. Laneuville O, Breuer DK, Xu N, et al. Fatty acid substrate specificities of human prostaglandin-endoperoxide H synthase-1 and -2. J Biol Chem. 1995;270:19330–6.
15. Laneuville O, Breuer DK, DeWitt DL, Hla T, Funk CD, Smith WL. Differential inhibition of human prostaglandin endoperoxide H synthases-1 and -2 by nonsteroidal anti-inflammatory drugs. J Pharm Exp Ther. 1994;271:927–34.
16. Garavito RM, Picot D, Loll PJ. The 3.1 Å X-ray crystal structure of the integral membrane enzyme prostaglandin H2 synthase-1. Adv Prostaglandin Thromboxane Leukotriene Res. 1995;23:99–103.

9 Risk of gastrointestinal side effects caused by non-steroid anti-inflammatory drugs (NSAIDs)

H. JICK

Non-experimental (epidemiological) observational studies are, in general, often difficult to conduct and interpret. This is particularly true of observational drug safety studies which involve drug exposure(s) as the major risk factor of interest. These studies generally require the identification of large study populations for which detailed information on drug exposure and clinical illnesses are available. In the past, such information had to be obtained by patient interview or questionnaire and ad hoc review of clinical charts, making studies expensive and time consuming. More recently, large automated clinical data resources have become available which allow identification of people with certain illnesses and provide a readily available long-term computer record of drugs prescribed prior to the onset of illnesses. In using such resources for drug safety research, it is first necessary to establish that the computer-recorded medical information is of satisfactory completeness and accuracy. The ability to review the case histories of a study illness is essential. When the necessary quality of the information has been confirmed, reliable studies may be conducted rapidly and at low cost. When the relevant clinical information is available proper epidemiological techniques are required in order to organize, analyse and interpret the information. When drug effects are the primary objective of a study, one must appreciate that in observational studies, patients are selected to receive the drug prescribed and inevitably persons who receive a particular drug are different in a number of ways from patients who receive alternative drugs or no drug. Often this 'selection bias' is not important in interpreting the results of a study, provided that differences among persons receiving different treatments are adjusted for in an analysis of the results. If such differences are important and unmeasurable, as is often the case, this may lead to distorted or biased results.

Another critical aspect of drug safety studies is that outcome illnesses rarely involve a single well defined entity. For example, upper gastrointestinal bleeding (UGIB) may originate in the oesophagus, stomach or duodenum, and the severity is variable. It may occur in persons with a history of peptic ulcer or other predisposing disease or those with no such history. Since NSAIDs are generally contraindicated in persons who are predisposed to UGIB, a study of the relationship between NSAID use and UGIB must take into account past medical history in the selection of subjects and thus appropriately deal with this issue.

The above considerations cover only a few of the technical aspects of conducting and interpreting observational drug studies. Unfortunately, it is necessary fully to appreciate proper epidemiological techniques to evaluate whether a given study provides reliable and interpretable results. Different studies which on the surface appear to evaluate the same research question, often provide conflicting results. While this may sometimes be due to chance, it is most often caused by differences in the quality and details of the methodology used.

The question which is addressed in this paper relates to the relationship between NSAID exposure and risk of UGIB. This subject has been addressed in over two dozen observational studies over the past 25 years. Bollini et al. reviewed 20 such studies in an article published in 1992[1]. Based on their understanding of generally accepted epidemiological principles, they judged that only eight (40%) of the studies used adequate methodology. Four of the studies estimated that the relative risk (RR) of UGIB when comparing NSAID users with non-users was between 1.0 and 2.0. In three studies the RR estimate was 2.1–4.0, and in one study the RR estimate was >4.0. These studies, primarily derived from paper-based information, evaluated different NSAIDs and had different criteria for the diagnosis of UGIB. This in part explains the apparent differences in the findings.

More recently, two large studies on this subject have been published, both of which applied technically sound, carefully defined methodology. The large amount of information available allowed risks to be estimated for many individual NSAIDs in relation to dose and duration of treatment, and the evaluation of numerous risk factors, other than NSAIDs, for UGIB. The first of these published studies[2] used a case–control design and was derived from a large UK-based computerized data resource, now known as The General Practice Research Database (GPRD). The quality and completeness of the information recorded in the GPRD (formerly known as VAMP Research) has been repeatedly documented[3-5]. The study encompassed 1457 well documented cases (aged 25–77 years) of UGIB or perforation and 10 000 randomly selected controls from the base population who were assigned a random index date. Persons with a history of predisposing conditions such as gastric cancer and chronic liver or renal disease were excluded from the study. A substantial number of independent risk factors for UGIB were recorded and controlled for by logistic regression. These included age, sex, smoking, calendar year and prior history of peptic ulcer disease. Adjusted relative risk estimates provided in the tables were derived from a logistic model controlling for these variables. Four NSAID exposure categories were evaluated.

Definition of NSAID exposure

A person was defined as a current NSAID user when the last NSAID prescription before the index date, i.e. the date of diagnosis of UGIB, was ordered during the previous month (a month's supply is the average dispensing duration of an NSAID prescription in the UK) or if the time from the date of the prescription to the index date was longer but the duration of therapy extended at least to the index date. Current use was subdivided into current single use (only one individual NSAID during the

150 days before the index date) and current multiple use (more than one individual NSAID during the 150 days before the index date).

An NSAID aggregate variable was created representing the use of any of the NSAIDs included in the study. The effect of dose was investigated for NSAIDs as a group and for four individual NSAIDs: sufficient information was available for stratification into low and high daily dose categories. Duration of use was defined as the number of consecutive prescriptions (following each other with a maximum interval of 90 days) among current single users. Duration was classified as 'unknown' when there was less than 6 months' history in the automated prescription file.

A person was defined as a recent past user when the last NSAID prescription before the index date was written 60–31 days before that date and the prescribed course of therapy finished before the index date. A person was defined as a past user when the last NSAID prescription before the index date was written 150–61 days before that date and the computer-recorded duration of therapy finished before the index date. Finally, a person was considered to be a non-user of NSAIDs if there was no prescription for an NSAID within 150 days of the index date.

RESULTS

Among the 1457 cases of UGIB, the site of the bleeding or perforation was gastric in 483 and duodenal in 787; 40 patients had multiple bleeding sites and for 147 'peptic ulcer' only was recorded. Perforation was reported in 261 cases. The relative risk of UGIB (Table 1) associated with all NSAID current use was 4.7 (see tables for 95% confidence intervals). The relative risk estimate was significantly higher for current multiple users (RR=9.0) than for current single users (RR=4.1). The risk was substantially lower for recent past users and that for past users was similar to the risk in non-users. Adjustment for current aspirin use did not substantially affect the results.

Other independent risk factors for UGIB were increasing age, male sex, smoking and history of ulcer (Table 1). The relative risks associated with NSAIDs were similar in the four age categories. We estimated the interaction between age and NSAID use, with people younger than 60 years and not exposed to NSAIDs as the reference group. The relative risk was 2.8 in people under 60 years of age exposed to NSAIDs, 3.7 in those of 60 years and older not exposed to NSAIDs, and 13.2 in those of 60 years and older exposed to NSAIDs. The relative risk associated with current NSAID use was slightly greater among women than men. Smoking increased the risk of UGIB by about 40%. The relative risk estimates associated with NSAID use were slightly greater for gastric than for duodenal bleeding and greater for perforation than for bleeding only.

Previous bleeding or perforation of the upper gastrointestinal tract was the single most important predictor of UGIB (relative risk 13.5). The relative risk of UGIB associated with NSAID use was higher in people without a history of peptic ulcer disease than in those with such a history. To examine the joint effect of exposure to NSAIDs and history of peptic ulcer we used as a common reference group people not currently exposed to NSAIDs and with no history of peptic ulcer (history of dyspepsia

Table 1   Relative risks of UGIB associated with various risk factors

	Cases (n = 1457)	Controls (n = 10 000)	Adjusted relative risk (95% CI)	
NSAID exposure				
No use	1106	9083	1	
All current use	241	365	4.7	(3.8 – 5.7)
single	194	318	4.1	(3.3 – 5.1)
multiple	47	47	9.0	(5.7 – 14.2)
Recent past use	44	169	1.9	(1.3 – 2.8)
Past use	66	383	1.4	(1.0 – 1.8)
Age (years)				
25 – 49	374	5561	1	
50 – 59	250	1740	1.6	(1.4 – 2.0)
60 – 69	376	1630	3.1	(2.5 – 3.7)
70 – 80	457	1069	5.6	(4.6 – 6.9)
Sex				
Male	958	5005	1	
Female	499	4995	0.5	(0.4 – 0.5)
Ulcer history				
No history	862	9017	1	
Dyspepsia	147	445	2.9	(2.4 – 3.6)
Ulcer without complication	278	433	6.1	(5.1 – 7.3)
Ulcer with complication	170	105	13.5	(10.3 – 17.7)
Use of other drugs[a]				
Oral corticosteroid use	38	64	2.2	(1.4 – 3.5)
Anticoagulant use	19	13	6.4	(2.8 – 14.6)

[a]Reference category was people who did not receive a prescription for relevant drugs within 5 months before index date

alone was not included). The relative risk was 5.4 for those exposed to NSAIDs only, 8.7 for those with a history of peptic ulcer only and 17.2 for those with both risk factors. In view of this effect on risk and the small number of people with a history of peptic ulcer, further analyses of the risk associated with NSAID use are presented for the subset of patients without history of peptic ulcer. The relative risk associated with NSAID current single use was significantly higher among those exposed to high doses than among those exposed to low doses (Table 2). With respect to duration, the relative risk after the first prescription (4.0) was no greater than the overall risk, and the risk increased slightly with long term therapy (Table 2).

There were important differences in the risk associated with the individual NSAIDs (Table 3). Azapropazone and piroxicam had relative risks >10. The five other NSAIDs assessed individually showed some variation in risk, but all had relative risks similar to that for overall NSAID use. Ibuprofen had the smallest risk. We were able to study a dose – effect relationship for four individual NSAIDs. Indomethacin and ibuprofen showed a substantial increase in risk from a low to a high daily dose (Table 3).

Table 2   Relative risk of UGIB associated with NSAID current single use[a]

	Cases (n = 862)	Controls (n = 9017)	Adjusted relative risk (95% CI)	
Daily dose				
No use	615	8222	1	
Low dose	45	150	2.6	(1.8 – 3.8)
High dose	90	118	7.0	(5.2 – 9.6)
Unknown	3	3	6.7	(1.2 – 37.4)
No. of NSAID prescriptions				
None	615	8222	1	
1	40	104	4.0	(2.7 – 6.1)
2 – 3	15	37	3.2	(1.7 – 6.1)
4 – 6	10	27	2.8	(1.3 – 6.0)
7 – 12	30	34	6.7	(3.9 – 11.4)
≥ 13	38	53	6.4	(4.0 – 10.2)
Unknown	5	16	3.5	(1.2 – 10.3)

[a]Only patients with no history of peptic ulcer were included

Table 3   Relative risk of UGIB associated with individual NSAIDs[a]

	Cases (n = 862)	Controls (n = 9017)	Adjusted relative risk (95% CI)	
NSAID current use				
No use	615	8222	1	
Ibuprofen	20	74	2.9	(1.7 – 5.0)
Other[b]	13	39	2.9	(1.5 – 5.6)
Naproxen	15	46	3.1	(1.7 – 5.9)
Diclofenac	25	53	3.9	(2.3 – 6.5)
Ketoprofen	14	20	5.4	(2.6 – 11.3)
Indomethacin	20	24	6.3	(3.3 – 12.2)
Multiple NSAIDs	33	43	8.9	(5.4 – 14.7)
Piroxicam	20	11	18.0	(8.2 – 39.6)
Azapropazone	11	4	23.4	(6.9 – 79.5)
Daily dose[c]				
None	615	8222	1	
Ibuprofen ≤ 1500 mg	12	59	2.1	(1.1 – 4.1)
Ibuprofen > 1500 mg	8	14	6.5	(2.6 – 16.4)
Naproxen ≤ 750 mg	5	14	4.0	(1.3 – 11.8)
Naproxen > 750 mg	10	31	3.1	(1.4 – 6.6)
Diclofenac < 100 mg	18	35	4.1	(2.2 – 7.6)
Diclofenac > 100 mg	7	18	3.4	(1.4 – 8.5)
Indomethacin ≤ 75 mg	3	15	1.4	(0.3 – 5.8)
Indomethacin > 75 mg	16	8	14.4	(5.7 – 36.4)

[a]Only patients with no history of peptic ulcer were included
[b]Mefenamic acid, fenbufen, fenoprofen, flurbiprofen, diflunisal, sulindac, tenoxicam, tiaprofenic acid, etodolac, and nabumetone
[c]Among current users of the four NSAIDs listed were four people with unknown daily dose

DISCUSSION

This study has confirmed that the use of NSAIDs is independently associated with an increased risk of UGIB. The excess risk of UGIB associated with NSAID use was similar irrespective of the site of bleeding, but the risk of perforation was somewhat greater than that of bleeding only. Both short and long duration of NSAID exposure increased the risk of UGIB. An adjustment for current aspirin use recorded on computer did not greatly alter our findings. Overall, there was a striking dose–response effect, and the increased risk associated with a high daily dose was independent of treatment duration. Similarly, people who had recently changed from one NSAID to another and/or received more than one NSAID simultaneously had more than twice the risk of individuals exposed to only one NSAID. The estimated risk in this group of multiple NSAID users was of the same magnitude as that among single NSAID users receiving a high daily dose.

History of peptic ulcer was not only the most important risk factor for the occurrence of an episode of UGIB but also an important effect modifier of the risk of UGIB associated with NSAIDs. Our estimated relative risk of UGIB associated with the use of NSAIDs was smaller in those with a history of peptic ulcer. However, since such patients are nine times more likely than others to develop UGIB, they are vulnerable to any further increase in risk due to NSAID exposure. We conclude that NSAIDs should be administered very cautiously to patients with a history of peptic ulcer.

The finding of low risk among users of ibuprofen is not new. However, the risk was substantially greater for those using a high dose than those on a low dose. Thus, the overall low risk associated with ibuprofen is largely accounted for by the estimate of risk in the low daily dose category, which accounted for most of the use (80%) in our study population.

Shortly after the publication of García Rodríguez and Jick study[2], another well designed large case–control study of NSAIDs and UGIB was published[6]. This study was based on patient interviews. The study population comprised 1144 cases of peptic ulcer bleeding (patients ≥60 years of age) and exposure to NSAIDs in the cases was compared with that in approximately equal numbers of hospital and neighbourhood controls matched to the cases on age and sex. Adjusted RR estimates for various NSAIDs were calculated using logistic regression to control for aspirin use, smoking, alcohol and previous peptic ulcer and/or dyspepsia.

The results of this study are closely similar to those of the García Rodríguez and Jick study[2]. Table 4 provides the results of the two latest studies together with rankings of individual NSAIDs derived from spontaneous anecdotal reports sent to the Committee on the Safety of Medicines (CSM)[7]. The CSM data are based on the number of reports received divided by the estimated sales of each NSAID[7].

Based on the best available evidence, it seems reasonable to conclude that the risk of UGIB is about four times higher for users of NSAIDs as a group compared with non-users of NSAIDs. In addition, there is now good evidence to suggest that the risk varies according to individual NSAID use and is dose-related for some NSAIDs. Ibuprofen at low doses appears to have the lowest risk, and azapropazone the highest risk. The risk for the remaining NSAIDs appears to be intermediate. Finally, it may

Table 4 *Odds ratio and 95% CI for bleeding and perforation[a] or acute gastrointestinal bleeding[b], and CSM rank order of serious reports of gut toxicity expressed per million prescriptions in the first 5 years of marketing*

	CSM ranking	García Rodríguez and Jick[a]		Langman et al.[b]	
		Ratio	95% CI	Ratio	95% CI
Overall		4.7	3.8–5.7	4.5	3.6–5.6
Ibuprofen	1	2.9	1.78–5.0	2.0	1.4–2.8
Diclofenac	2	3.9	2.3–6.5	4.2	2.6–6.8
Naproxen	5	3.1	1.7–5.9	9.1	5.5–15.1
Ketoprofen	6	5.4	2.6–11.3	23.7	7.6–74.2
Indomethacin	c	6.3	3.3–12.2	11.3	6.3–20.3
Piroxicam	11	18.0	8.2–39.6	13.7	7.1–26.3
Azapropazone	12	23.4	6.9–79.5	31.5	10.3–96.9

[c]Not ranked by CSM. Marketed before yellow card scheme

be concluded that NSAIDs should be used with special caution in persons with other risk factors for UGIB. These include the elderly, males, those with a prior history of peptic ulcer disease and cigarette smokers. NSAIDs should also be used with caution in persons who are heavy users of alcohol and those who are receiving anticoagulants and steroids.

References

1. Bollini P, García Rodríguez LA, Pérez Gutthann S, Walker AM. The impact of research quality and study design on epidemiologic estimates of the effect of nonsteroidal anti-inflammatory drugs on upper gastrointestinal tract disease. Arch Intern Med. 1992;152:1289–95.
2. García Rodríguez LA, Jick H. Risk of upper gastrointestinal bleeding and perforation associated with individual non-steroidal anti-inflammatory drugs. Lancet. 1994;343:769–72.
3. Jick H, Jick SS, Derby LE. Validation of information recorded on general practitioner based computerised data resource in the United Kingdom. Br Med J. 1991;302:766–8.
4. Jick H, Terris BZ, Derby LE, Jick SS. Further validation of information recorded on a general practitioner based computerized data resource in the United Kingdom. Pharmacoepidemiol Drug Safety. 1992;1:347–9.
5. Jick H, Jick SS, Gurewich V, Myers MW, Vasilakis C. Risk of idiopathic cardiovascular death and nonfatal venous thromboembolism in women using oral contraceptives with differing progestagen components. Lancet. 1995;346:1589–93.
6. Langman MJS, Weil J, Wainwright P et al. Risks of bleeding peptic ulcer associated with individual non-steroidal anti-inflammatory drugs. Lancet. 1994;343:1075–8.
7. Bateman DN. NSAIDs: time to re-evaluate gut toxicity. Lancet. 1994;343:1051–2.

10 Expression and regulation of cyclooxygenase-2 in synovial tissues of arthritic patients

L. J. CROFFORD

Rheumatoid arthritis (RA) is a systemic inflammatory disease, the dominant clinical feature of which is symmetrical polyarticular synovitis. Characteristic histo-pathological changes include infiltration of synovial tissues with mononuclear inflammatory cells, marked proliferation of synovial lining cells and sub-lining fibroblast-like cells and genesis of new supporting blood vessels. Inflammation of synovial tissue causes pain and swelling of joints. Proliferative synovia erode articular cartilage and juxta-articular bone. Although the aetiology of RA is not known, the pathogenesis involves complex interactions between cells of the immune system and resident cells of the synovia. A number of mediators, including cytokines, growth factors and eicosanoids, produced by infiltrating mononuclear cells as well as by endothelial cells and fibroblast-like cells (synoviocytes), contribute to the proliferative and invasive phenotype of inflamed synovial tissues in RA.

Aspirin and non-steroid anti-inflammatory drugs (NSAIDs) are used extensively in the treatment of RA and other inflammatory diseases[1]. It was established by Vane and colleagues that aspirin and other NSAIDs inhibit cyclooxygenase (COX, PGH synthase), the central enzyme in the prostaglandin (PG) synthetic pathway[2]. PG levels are elevated in the synovial fluids and synovial tissues of patients with RA. Levels of synovial fluid PGs, including PGE_2, TXB_2, $PGF_{2\alpha}$, and 6-keto $PGF_{1\alpha}$, decrease after treatment with NSAIDs[3]. PGs are thought to be important autocrine and paracrine mediators of inflammation in RA, and may play a role in the erosion of juxta-articular bone by induction of matrix metalloproteinases[4]. However, the in vivo effect of increased PG levels in joint tissues is likely to be pleiotropic; for example, inhibition of PG production exacerbates cartilage erosion, but reduces bone loss[5].

There are two isoforms of COX, COX-1 and COX-2. COX-1 is constitutively expressed in a wide range of cells and tissues[6], and may undergo slow changes in levels of expression associated with cellular differentiation[7]. COX-2 expression is highly regulated in vitro in response to many extracellular stimuli: it is increased dramatically by cytokines and mitogens and decreased by glucocorticoids[8,9]. The characteristics of COX-1 and -2 expression suggest that COX-1 may be the isoform important for production of PGs mediating homeostatic functions, while COX-2 may play a major role in increasing PG production in specific tissues affected by inflammatory pathology[8,10]. Specific inhibition of COX-2 may be useful in RA for more effective inhibition of localized PG production, since side effects might not limit dose. More complete understanding of molecular mechanisms responsible for the regulation of COX-2 in synovial tissues may also suggest alternative methods for decreasing COX-2 expression or function.

In this review, the available data regarding expression and regulation of COX-2 in synovial tissues are summarized. We will speculate on the role of COX-2 in the pathogenesis of the inflammatory synovitis of RA and the potential for COX-2 inhibitors in the treatment of chronic inflammatory arthritis.

COX EXPRESSION IN ANIMAL MODELS OF ARTHRITIS

Sano and colleagues evaluated expression of COX in joint tissues of Lewis rats over time after intraperitoneal injection of streptococcal cell walls (SCW) or intradermal injection of Freund's complete adjuvant[11]. These animal studies were performed prior to the characterization of the COX-2 isoform, and the antisera used recognizes both COX-1 and COX-2. Nevertheless, there was little immunostaining for COX in untreated animals, and markedly increased expression of immunoreactive COX that paralleled clinical arthritis. COX immunostaining was detected in multiple cell types within the joints and surrounding tissues, including synovial lining cells, sub-lining synovial fibroblast-like cells, vascular endothelial cells, infiltrating mononuclear inflammatory cells, chondrocytes, subchondral osteoblasts and adjacent bone marrow. In acute, non-T cell-dependent SCW-induced arthritis, treatment with the synthetic glucocorticoid dexamethasone decreased COX expression in a dose-dependent manner, while treatment with progesterone had no effect. Continuous infusion of dexamethasone in animals injected with adjuvant also suppressed expression of COX. Finally, although immunoreactive COX expression was markedly increased, there was no increase in COX-1 mRNA by reverse transcription and polymerase chain reaction (RT-PCR) analysis. The RT-PCR findings and the glucocorticoid sensitivity of the COX immunostaining strongly suggest that increased expression of COX-2 was responsible for the majority of the increased in vivo COX expression detected in these animal models of arthritis.

Anderson and co-workers performed specific COX isoform analysis of rats with adjuvant-induced arthritis[12]. They confirmed that COX-2, but not COX-1, mRNA increased concomitant with, or just prior to, the onset of detectable paw swelling. Increased expression of COX-2 mRNA was followed by increased COX-2 protein expression and tissue PGE_2 levels. Furthermore, treatment of arthritic animals with the specific COX-2 inhibitor SC-58125 (Searle, St Louis, MO) suppressed paw swelling by 80–85%. This level of suppression was equivalent to indomethacin, while dexamethasone inhibited paw oedema by 95–100%[12].

COX EXPRESSION IN SYNOVIA OF PATIENTS WITH RA AND OA

Using a polyclonal antibody that recognized both COX-1 and COX-2, Sano and colleagues examined synovial tissues from patients with RA or osteoarthritis (OA) and from non-arthritic patients with traumatic injury for COX expression by immunohistochemical staining[11]. Synovial tissues from patients with RA exhibited intense staining of the synovial lining layer, sub-synovial synoviocytes, vascular

Table 1   Regulation of COX-2 in synoviocytes in vitro

Increased by
   Phorbol ester, lipopolysaccharide
   IL-1β, TNF-α, TGF-β; not IL-6
   Superantigen in IFN-γ-stimulated cells
Decreased by
   Dexamethasone
   IL-4

endothelial cells and mononuclear inflammatory cells. The extent and intensity of COX immunostaining correlated with the degree of mononuclear cell infiltration that provided a measure of the synovial inflammation. COX immunostaining was less intense in patients with OA, and little immunoreactive COX was detected in non-arthritic synovial tissues.

An antibody specific for the unique carboxy-terminal peptide of human COX-2 was generated and used for immunostaining of rheumatoid synovial tissues[8]. Staining for COX-2 using specific antisera was far more variable than immunohistochemical staining using the polyclonal anti-COX antisera[8,11]. While there was staining in vascular endothelial cells and infiltrating mononuclear inflammatory cells, there was little staining in the synovial lining layer and sub-lining synoviocytes. In addition, levels of COX-2 mRNA were lower than those of COX-1 mRNA in these patients by RT-PCR analysis[8]. The lower levels of COX-2 in patients may be due to the more rapid degradation of COX-2 mRNA than that of the more stable COX-1 transcript[13].

COX EXPRESSION AND REGULATION IN SYNOVIAL TISSUES IN VITRO

In vitro analysis of cultured human synovial tissues has contributed to the understanding of factors that regulate expression of COX (Table 1). We evaluated the expression and regulation of COX-1 and COX-2 polypeptide in fresh explants of rheumatoid synovia[8]. These synovial explant tissues contain macrophage-like and fibroblast-like synovial cells, as well as endothelial cells and mononuclear inflammatory cells. COX-1 and COX-2 were detected by immunoprecipitation of metabolically labelled proteins and/or by Western blot under basal conditions. Treatment with interleukin (IL)-1β or phorbol ester (PMA) markedly increased expression of COX-2, and pretreatment with dexamethasone eliminated basal and stimulated COX-2 expression. These same treatments had no effect on the level of COX-1 expression.

Since synoviocytes are a major source of PG in rheumatoid synovial tissues, we examined expression and regulation of COX mRNA and polypeptide expression in primary cultured rheumatoid synoviocytes[8]. COX-2 polypeptide was not expressed at baseline, but was present after treatment with IL-1β and PMA. IL-1β-stimulated expression was completely inhibited by pretreatment with dexamethasone. A small amount of COX-2 mRNA was present at baseline, and its expression paralleled that of polypeptide in response to all treatments. Hulkower and colleagues also demonstrated that levels of COX-2 mRNA and polypeptide in rheumatoid synoviocytes increase after treatment with IL-1β[9]. These authors also demonstrated coordinately increased expression of $cPLA_2$ mRNA and polypeptide in RA synoviocytes. PGE_2 levels increased after induction of these synthetic enzymes[9].

Treatment with the transcription inhibitor actinomycin-D completely eliminated basal and stimulated COX-2 mRNA expression; treatment with cycloheximide, which inhibits translation, markedly increased COX-2 expression[8]. These findings are consistent with the notion that COX-2 acts as an immediate-early gene in these cells. COX-1 mRNA was not affected by any of these treatments.

Mehindate and co-workers examined regulation of COX-2 in rheumatoid synoviocytes in a system whereby synoviocytes were induced to express MHC class II by treatment with interferon (IFN)-γ, then exposed to superantigen cross-linked with antibody[4]. Expression of COX-2, but not COX-1, was increased after exposure to superantigen. Induction of COX-2, as well as $cPLA_2$, was associated with increased expression of PGE_2 and expression of increased collagenase, the matrix metalloproteinase implicated in tissue destruction in inflammatory and erosive joint diseases such as RA. Increased collagenase gene expression could be inhibited with indomethacin and arachidonyl-trifluoromethyl-ketone, an inhibitor of $cPLA_2$[4].

A recent report by Sugiyama and colleagues demonstrated that IL-4 inhibited the spontaneous production of PGE_2 in freshly isolated synovial cells[14]. IL-4 also antagonized LPS- and IL-1-stimulated increases in levels of COX-2, but not COX-1, polypeptide and mRNA. In support of a role for IL-4 in the suppression of COX-2, both IL-4 and IL-13 inhibited IL-1-induced COX-2, but not COX-1, mRNA expression and PGE_2 production in cultured murine osteoblasts[15].

TRANSCRIPTIONAL AND POST-TRANSCRIPTIONAL REGULATION OF COX-2 mRNA

The promoter/enhancer of the human COX-2 gene contains a number of potential binding sites for recognized transcription factors (Figure 1). Several of these transcription factors are known to be stimulated by pro-inflammatory cytokines, including nuclear factor-κB (NF-κB), CCAAT/enhancer binding protein (C/EBP, also known as nuclear factor for IL-6 or NF-IL6) and the cyclic AMP responsive element binding protein (CREBP) (Figure 1). We have found that NF-κB plays a role in early induction of COX-2 in human rheumatoid synoviocytes (unpublished data). Hempel and co-workers demonstrated that LPS-stimulated COX-2 expression in human alveolar macrophages can be inhibited by changes in oxidant tone, a manipulation known to inhibit NF-κB. In mouse 3T3 fibroblasts, the v-*src* oncogene, which acts as a protein tyrosine kinase, stimulates COX-2 expression through the CRE transcriptional response element[16]. In a rat granulosa cell system, Sirois and Richards showed that stimulation of COX-2 transcription by gonadotropins utilized C/EBPβ[17]. Inoue and co-workers also demonstrated the importance of the C/EBP family of transcription factors in the up-regulation of COX-2 expression in bovine or human vascular endothelial cells stimulated with lipopolysaccharide and phorbol

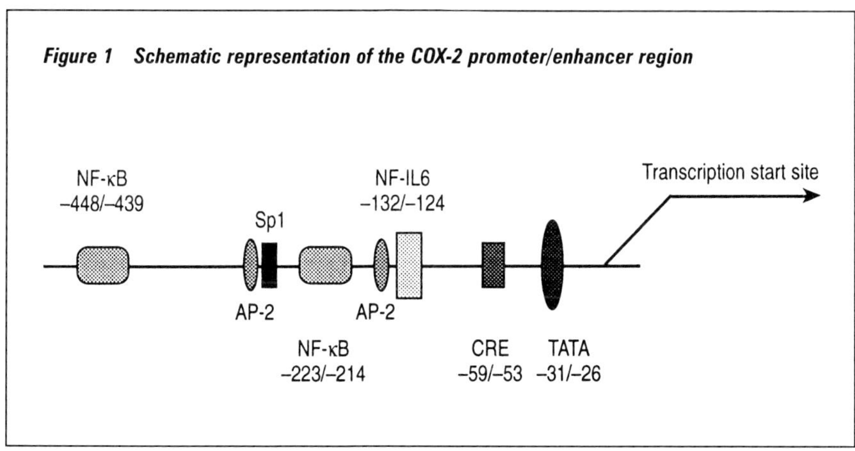

Figure 1 Schematic representation of the COX-2 promoter/enhancer region

ester[18]. In their studies, C/EBP bound to both the NF-IL6 and CRE sites in the COX-2 promoter, and c/EBPδ appeared to be the most important isoform in stimulating transcription[18]. The CRE of the human COX 2 gene is an asymmetrical CRE site of the type that has been shown to bind heterodimers of C/EBP and CREBP[19]. Finally, C/EBP has also been shown to complex with the p50 subunit of NF-κB[20].

The COX-2 transcript contains multiple copies of the 'AUUA' mRNA instability sequence characteristic of many cytokine-responsive mRNAs with a high rate of degradation[21]. These unstable transcripts are also induced by inhibitors of translation, possibly by blocking synthesis of an mRNA degradation factor(s). Studies by Ristimaki and co-workers demonstrated a COX-2 mRNA half-life of 1 h in cells pretreated with cycloheximide[13]. IL-1 treatment prolonged the half-life of COX-2 mRNA, and this effect was potentiated when transcription was inhibited[13].

POTENTIAL ROLE FOR COX-2 IN THE PATHOGENESIS OF RA

Locally increased PG levels may play a role in both acute and chronic inflammatory processes (Figure 2). Increased COX-2 expression appears to be an important enzymatic determinant of increased PG production in acute inflammation, as demonstrated by the ability of selective COX-2 inhibitors to block carrageenan-induced inflammation when administered prior to the stimulus and to significantly decrease inflammatory indices and PG levels when administered 6 h after an acute inflammatory stimulus[22]. A role for COX-2 in more chronic inflammatory processes is suggested by the increased COX-2 expression seen in adjuvant-induced arthritis in rats. Selective COX-2 inhibitors are able to decrease paw swelling substantially in this model of chronic inflammation[12]. Nevertheless, the role played by PGs in the development and maintenance of chronic inflammatory arthritis is quite complex, with some effects likely to contribute to ongoing inflammation and other effects likely to inhibit leukocyte functions[23].

The chronically inflamed synovial tissues of patients with RA display

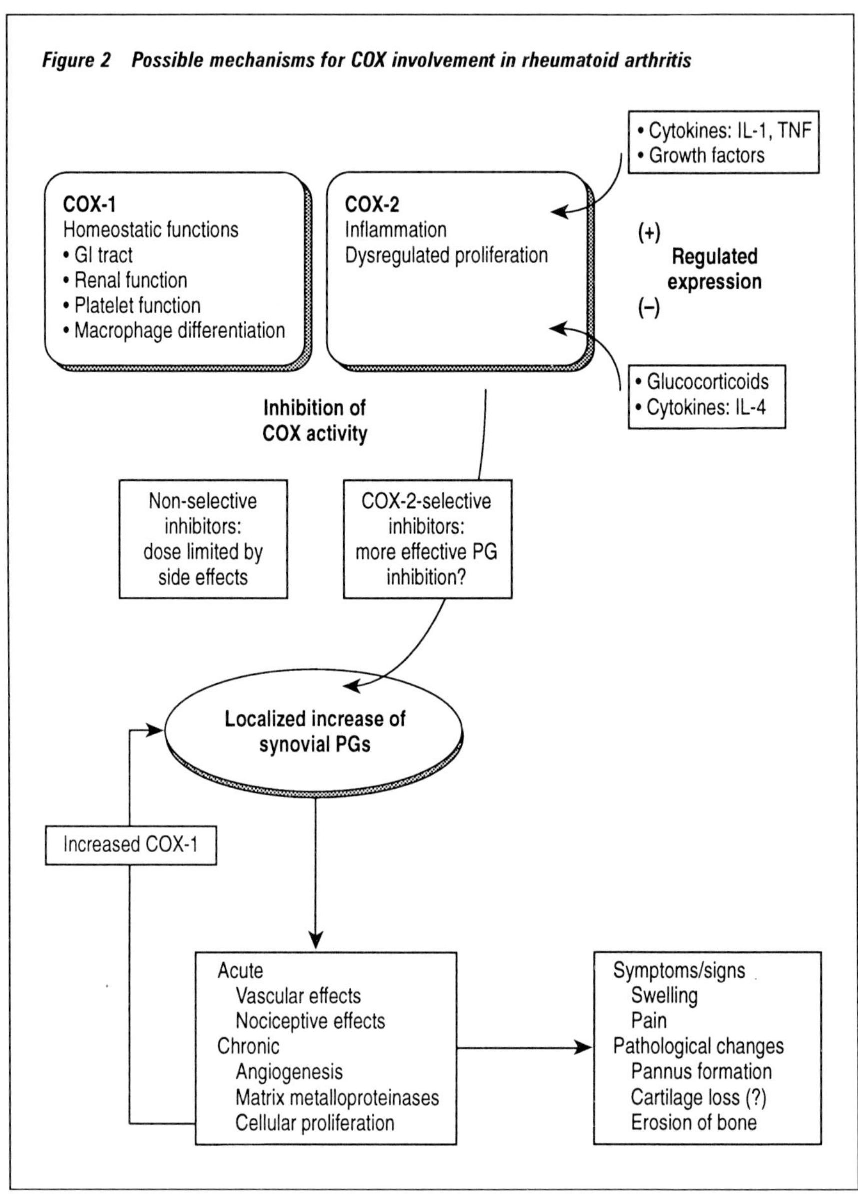

characteristics often associated with malignancies, including proliferation, angiogenesis and invasion of surrounding tissues[24,25]. This 'transformed' phenotype is not constitutive, however, but appears to be mediated by locally elaborated factors, including cytokines, growth factors and eicosanoids. Interactions between resident cells of the synovia and infiltrating mononuclear inflammatory cells appear to be a key factor in the development and maintenance of this phenotype, in part by production of cytokine mediators[26]. Increased COX-2 expression and PG production could play a role in the 'transformed' phenotype exhibited by rheumatoid synovial tissues. Tsujii and DuBois demonstrated that stable over-expression of COX-2 increases resistance of rat intestinal epithelial cells to apoptosis[27]. PGs are important mediators of matrix metalloproteinase expression by synoviocytes, and increased COX-2 expression has been implicated in vitro as correlating with stimulated increases in collagenase[4]. PGs may contribute to the angiogenesis that is required to support synoviocyte proliferation and pannus formation. COX-2 expression is increased by pro-inflammatory cytokines in human vascular endothelial cells, making a role for COX-2 in the angiogenesis associated with rheumatoid synovia plausible[13]. However, since there is likely to be an overall increase in COX-1 levels in rheumatoid synovial tissues due to markedly increased cellularity, the relative role of COX-2 in maintaining PG levels in chronic inflammatory conditions is uncertain[8,11].

POTENTIAL ROLE OF SPECIFIC COX-2 INHIBITORS IN RA

Glucocorticoids exhibit selective effects on COX-2, compared with COX-1; however, glucocorticoids affect the metabolism of arachidonic acid at multiple levels[1,8]. In addition, glucocorticoids have effects on multiple inflammatory processes mediated directly through the glucocorticoid receptor. The synovitis of RA is exquisitely sensitive to corticosteroids. There are data to suggest that patients with RA may produce insufficient glucocorticoids[28], which could contribute to inappropriately sustained expression of COX-2. Recent reports have suggested that low-dose glucocorticoids, in combination with other treatments, in patients with a disease duration of <2 years may reduce radiographic progression of disease[29]. How these findings may relate to glucocorticoid effects on COX-2 expression is not known.

Selective non-steroid COX-2 inhibitors are unlikely to be as effective as glucocorticoids in the treatment of RA. There are theoretical and experimental reasons to believe, however, that selective pharmacological inhibitors of COX-2 have a more favourable side effect profile than NSAIDs currently in use, which inhibit both COX-1 and COX-2. Selective COX-2 inhibitors should decrease PG production in situations where COX-2 activity is increased, but should not alter basal PG production mediated via COX-1. This is likely to result in less pronounced effects on tissues where PGs mediate important homeostatic functions, including the gastrointestinal tract, kidney and platelets. In experiments performed by Masferrer and colleagues, NS-398, a selective COX-2 inhibitor, suppressed PG production in inflamed tissues, but did not inhibit gastric PG synthesis. These results stand in sharp contrast to results with indomethacin, which inhibited both lesional and gastric PG production, and caused gastric damage[22]. Furthermore, preliminary data from Bjarnason and colleagues showed fewer gastric erosions in osteoarthritis patients taking a selective COX-2 inhibitor, flosulide, than in those receiving naproxen[30]. These data suggest that doses of selective COX-2 inhibitors that may more completely suppress local production of PGs in synovial tissues could be used in patients with inflammatory arthritis. Evaluation of selective COX-2 inhibition for effects on symptoms and progression of destructive synovitis may yield clues relating to the role of the COX-2 in RA.

References

1. Abramson SB, Weissman G. The mechanisms of action of nonsteroidal antiinflammatory drugs. Arthritis Rheum. 1989;32:1–9.
2. Vane JR. Inhibition of prostaglandin synthesis as a mechanism of action for aspirin-like drugs. Nature. 1971;231:232–5.
3. Day RO, Francis H, Vial J, Geisslinger G, Williams KM. Naproxen concentrations in plasma and synovial fluid and effects on prostanoid concentrations. J Rheumatol. 1995;22:2295–303.
4. Mehindate K, Al-Daccak R, Dayer J-M et al. Superantigen-induced collagenase gene expression in human IFN-γ-treated fibroblast-like synoviocytes involves prostaglandin E_2. J Immunol. 1995;155:3570–7.
5. Vane JR, Mitchell JA, Appleton I et al. Inducible isoforms of cyclooxygenase and nitric-oxide synthase in inflammation. Proc Natl Acad Sci USA. 1994;91:2046–50.
6. Funk CD, Funk LB, Kennedy ME, Pong AS, Fitzgerald GA. Human platelet/erythroleukemia cell prostaglandin G/H synthase: cDNA cloning, expression, and gene chromosomal assignment. FASEB J. 1991;5:2304–12.
7. Smith CJ, Morrow JD, Roberts LJ, Marnett LJ. Differentiation of monocytoid THP-1 cells with phorbol ester induces expression of prostaglandin endoperoxide synthase-1 (COX-1). Biochem Biophys Res Commun. 1993;192:787–93.
8. Crofford LJ, Wilder RL, Ristimaki AP, Remmers EF, Epps HR, Hla T. Cyclooxygenase-1 and -2 expression in rheumatoid synovial tissues: effects of interleukin-1β, phorbol ester, and corticosteroids. J Clin Invest. 1994;93:1095–101.
9. Hulkower KI, Wertheimer SJ, Levin W et al. Interleukin-1β induces cytosolic phospholipase A2 and prostaglandin H synthase in rheumatoid synovial fibroblasts. Evidence for their roles in the production of prostaglandin E_2. Arthritis Rheum. 1994;37:653–61.
10. Crofford LJ. Expression and regulation of COX-2 in synovial tissues of arthritis patients. In: Vane J, Botting J, Botting R, eds. Improved Non-Steroid Anti-inflammatory Drugs. COX-2 Enzyme Inhibitors. London: Kluwer Academic Publishers and William Harvey Press; 1996: 133–43.
11. Sano H, Hla T, Maier JAM et al. In vivo cyclooxygenase expression in synovial tissues of patients with rheumatoid arthritis and osteoarthritis and rats with adjuvant and streptococcal cell wall arthritis. J Clin Invest. 1992;89:97–108.
12. Anderson GD, Hauser SD, Bremer ME, McGarity KL, Isakson PC, Gregory SA. Selective inhibition of cyclooxygenase-2 reverses inflammation and expression of COX-2 and IL-6 in rat adjuvant arthritis. J Clin Invest. In press.
13. Ristimaki A, Garfinkel S, Wessendorf J, Maciag T, Hla T. Induction of cyclooxygenase-2 by interleukin-1 alpha. Evidence for post-transcriptional regulation. J Biol Chem. 1994;269:11769–75.
14. Sugiyama E, Taki H, Kuroda A, Mino T, Hori T, Kobayashi M. Interleukin-4 inhibits prostaglandin E_2 production by freshly prepared rheumatoid synovial cells via inhibition of biosynthesis and gene expression of cyclooxygenase II but not those of cyclooxygenase I. Arthritis Rheum. 1995;38(suppl):S352.
15. Onoe Y, Miyaura C, Kaminakayashiki T et al. IL-13 and IL-4 inhibit bone resorption by suppressing cyclooxygenase-2-dependent prostaglandin synthesis in osteoblasts. J Immunol. 1996;156:758–64.
16. Xie W, Fletcher BS, Andersen RD, Herschman HR. v-*src* induction of the TIS10/PGS2 prostaglandin synthase gene is mediated by an ATF/CRE transcription response element. Mol Cell Biol. 1994;14:6531–9.
17. Sirois J, Richards JS. Transcription regulation of the rat prostaglandin endoperoxide synthase 2 gene in granulosa cells: Evidence for the role of a *cis*-acting C/EBPβ promoter element. J Biol Chem. 1993;268:21931–8.
18. Inoue H, Yokoyama C, Hara S, Tone Y, Tanabe T. Transcriptional regulation of human prostaglandin-endoperoxide synthase-2 gene by lipopolysaccharide and phorbol ester in vascular endothelial cells. J Biol Chem. 1995;270:24965–71.

19. Tsukada J, Saito K, Waterman W, Webb AC, Auron PE. Transcription factors NF-IL6 and CREB recognize a common essential site in the human prointerleukin 1β gene. Mol Cell Biol. 1994; 14:7285–97.
20. LeClair KP, Blanar MA, Sharp PA. The p50 subunit of NF-κB associates with the NF-IL6 transcription factor. Proc Natl Acad Sci USA. 1992;89:8145–9.
21. Shaw G, Kamen R. A conserved AU sequence from the 3′ untranslated region of GM-CSF mRNA mediates selective mRNA degradation. Cell. 1986;29:659–7.
22. Masferrer JL, Zweifel BS, Manning PT et al. Selective inhibition of inducible cyclooxygenase 2 in vivo is antiinflammatory and nonulcerogenic. Proc Natl Acad Sci USA. 1994;91:3228–32.
23. Weissmann G. Prostaglandins as modulators rather than mediators of inflammation. J Lipid Mediators. 1993;6:275–86.
24. Brinckerhoff DR, Harris ED Jr. Survival of rheumatoid synovium implanted into nude mice. Am J Pathol. 1981;103:411–18.
25. Lafyatis R, Remmers EF, Roberts AB, Yocum DE, Sporn MB, Wilder RL. Anchorage-independent growth of synoviocytes from arthritic and normal joints: Stimulation by exogenous platelet derived growth factor and inhibition by transforming growth factor-beta and retinoids. J Clin Invest. 1989;83:1267–76.
26. Arend WP, Dayer J-M. Cytokines and cytokine inhibitors or antagonists in rheumatoid arthritis. Arthritis Rheum. 1990;33:305–15.
27. Tsujii M, DuBois RN. Alterations in cellular adhesion and apoptosis in epithelial cells overexpressing prostaglandin endoperoxide synthase 2. Cell. 1995;83:493–501.
28. Chikanza IC, Petrou P, Kingsley G, Chrousos G, Panayi GS. Defective hypothalamic response to immune and inflammatory stimuli in patients with rheumatoid arthritis. Arthritis Rheum. 1991; 35:1281–8.
29. Kirwan JR. The effect of glucocorticoids on joint destruction in rheumatoid arthritis. N Engl J Med. 1995;333:142–6.
30. Bjarnason I, Macpherson A, Schupp J, Hayllar J. A randomised, double-blind, crossover comparative endoscopy study on the tolerability of flosulide, a selective cyclo-oxygenase-2 inhibitor, and naproxen. Arthritis Rheum. 1995;38(suppl):S280.

11 Differential target tissue presentation and COX-2/COX-1 inhibition by non-steroid anti-inflammatory drugs: a rationale for a new classification

H. FENNER

INTRODUCTION

'Selecting a non-steroid anti-inflammatory drug (NSAID) for an individual patient remains more an art than a science'[1]. Prescribing of NSAIDs has been influenced by a lack of reliable scientific data on individual agents with respect to gastrointestinal (GI) tolerability or detrimental effects on cartilage metabolism. This has led to a number of unsubstantiated marketing claims about NSAIDs.

Reports that 'there are differences among NSAIDs and rational ways to distinguish their use in rheumatoid arthritis and other rheumatic diseases'[2] have not changed prescribing of NSAIDs, particularly as the causes of variation in patient response are poorly understood[3,4]. Differences in the pharmacokinetics of NSAIDs have not been used as selection criteria for prescribing NSAIDs. The relationship between half-life and the safety profile of NSAIDs is unclear, although a long half-life may be associated with a persistent effect on prostaglandin formation and function in the GI mucosa and kidney.

Clinical trials have failed to demonstrate significant differences in efficacy of currently available NSAIDs. This may in part be due to difficulties in objective clinical assessment of signs and symptoms of inflammation and the small sample size used in many studies. Differences in the safety profile of NSAIDs are therefore difficult to demonstrate for statistical reasons in the clinical development of a new agent, whereas post-marketing surveillance studies which include more patients, and pharmacoepidemiological studies, have indicated a higher gut toxicity of some agents.

The recent discovery of two distinct isoforms of cyclooxygenase (COX) has provided a convincing pharmacological rationale for variations in the efficacy and safety profile of NSAIDs. Prostanoids derived from the constitutive COX (COX-1) pathway regulate gut mucosal and kidney function and integrity, therefore inhibition of COX-1 may have detrimental effects. In contrast, COX-2 is only induced during inflammation. Agents which inhibit COX-2 down-regulate the mediators of inflammation and therefore have anti-inflammatory effects.

The tissue distribution of COX activity (relevant to arthritis) is different for the two isoforms. COX-2 activity is expressed in synovial cells; COX-1 activity is expressed in thrombocytes, gastrointestinal mucosa, and the kidney.

Differences in selectivity towards one of the two isoforms of the enzyme have been demonstrated for most of the currently available NSAIDs in various experimental systems including cell lines expressing human COX-1 and COX-2. Results of these studies, together with clinical data, provide evidence that agents with selectivity towards COX-2 have considerable safety advantages compared to those with selectivity towards COX-1 or compounds equipotent on COX-1 and COX-2. Research into new NSAIDs has demonstrated an improved risk/benefit profile in animal models of inflammation and ulcerogenicity of agents showing selective inhibition towards COX-2, e.g. meloxicam[5] and flosulide[6]. For example, the therapeutic ratio for meloxicam derived from the ID_{50} for inhibition of paw swelling in the adjuvant arthritis rat model and the ED_{50} for ulcerogenic effects on the rat stomach is 20, whereas for standard NSAIDs (naproxen and indomethacin) ratios of between 0.9 and 3.5 were found in the same experimental models. These results clearly indicate that it is possible to maintain anti-inflammatory activity and reduce the propensity for adverse effects on the GI system.

Pharmacokinetic and pharmacodynamic variables are important in determining the efficacy and safety profile of NSAIDs. Pharmacokinetic variables govern the relative distribution of the NSAIDs in the different compartments expressing the COX isoforms, while pharmacodynamic variables express the relative selectivity of the NSAID for COX-1 and COX-2. The present review will discuss the pharmacokinetic and pharmacodynamic data relating to a range of NSAIDs and will present the rationale behind a new system of classifying NSAIDs.

DIFFERENTIAL DISTRIBUTION OF NSAIDs INTO THE SYNOVIAL AND EXTRA-SYNOVIAL COMPARTMENT

The synovial fluid/plasma concentration/time course can be assessed after drug administration and is a measure of the relative NSAID concentration in the two compartments. A high ratio reflects the potential for synovial COX-2 inhibition and if the IC_{50} for COX-2 is low, this indicates potent anti-inflammatory activity. In contrast, a low synovial fluid/plasma ratio means higher drug concentrations in tissues where COX-1 is expressed. If the IC_{50} for COX-1 is low, then more pronounced effects on the GI mucosa and kidney may occur. Thus, a high ratio for synovial fluid/plasma concentration coupled with a low IC_{50} for COX-2 should be the preferred combination in terms of efficacy and tolerability.

The synovial fluid/plasma ratio of a NSAID is determined by physicochemical and pharmacokinetic parameters. Data relating to a number of NSAIDs are illustrated in Table 1. NSAIDs with a short plasma elimination half-life (1–3 h), e.g. indomethacin, have low ratios in the first hours after drug administration (at the time of maximal plasma concentrations) after which the ratios increase.

NSAIDs with an intermediate half-life, such as naproxen, show smaller fluctuations in the synovial fluid/plasma ratio: 0.36 at maximal plasma levels after 1.9 hours and 0.78 after 12 hours with a mean of 0.66 at steady state plasma levels (500 mg bid).

Table 1   Pharmacokinetic profile of NSAIDs

	C_{max} plasma μg/ml (hours)	C_{min} plasma μg/ml (hours)	C_{mean} plasma μg/ml (hours)	C_{max} synovial fluid μg/ml (hours)	C_{min} synovial fluid μg/ml (hours)	C_{mean} synovial fluid μg/ml (hours)	$C_{synovial\ fluid}/C_{plasma}$ at $C_{max\ plasma}$ (hours)	$C_{synovial\ fluid}/C_{plasma}$ at $C_{min\ plasma}$ (hours)	$C_{synovial\ fluid}/C_{plasma}$ at $C_{mean\ plasma}$	Reference
Diclofenac 50 mg	800×10^{-3} (3)	60×10^{-3} (8)		280×10^{-3} (3)	170×10^{-3} (8)		0.35 (3)	2.8 (8)		Fowler et al. 1983[7]
100 mg CR md			$220-110\times10^{-3}$ (4–8)			180×10^{-3} (4–8)			0.8	Fowler et al. 1986[8]
Indomethacin 50 mg	2.9 (1)	0.34 (9)	0.6–0.4 (3–7)	0.69 (2)	0.4 (9)	0.6–0.5 (3–7)	0.12 (1)	1.2 (9)		Emori et al. 1983[9]
Ibuprofen 600 mg repeated doses (day 3)	46 (1.3)	5 (7)	24 (3)	12 (3)	6 (7)		0.5 (1.3)	1.2 (7)		Gallo et al. 1986[10]
Naproxen 500 mg bid (day 7)	89 (1.9)	41 (12)	63	47 (5.2)	32 (12)	41	0.36 (1.9)	0.78 (12)	0.66	Day 1995[11]
Meloxicam 15 mg (steady state)	1.9 (5)	1.4 (24)		1.0 (5)	0.6 (24)		0.53 (5)	0.43 (24)	0.48	Degner et al. 1995[12]
Piroxicam 20 mg (steady state)	8.0 (3)	4.5 (24)		5.5 (3)	3.0 (24)		0.7 (3)	0.7 (24)	0.7	Kurowski et al. 1988[13]

Table 2   *Experimental models for the study of differential COX-2/COX-1 inhibition*

Whole cell assays	Human monocytes (whole blood assays): LPS-stimulated for COX-2
	Guinea pig peritoneal macrophages: unstimulated for COX-1, LPS-stimulated for COX-2
	Mouse peritoneal macrophages: unstimulated for COX-1, LPS-stimulated for COX-2
	Cultured bovine aortic endothelial cells (COX-1)
	LPS-stimulated J774.2 macrophages (mouse) (COX-2)
Cell lines expressing human COX-1 and COX-2	Cultured Cos-A2 cells (African green monkey kidney cells), transfected with human recombinant COX-1 and COX-2 (Baculovirus expression system)
Cell homogenates (broken cells)	Homogenate from cultured bovine aortic endothelial cells (COX-1)
	LPS-stimulated J774.2 macrophages (COX-2)
	Microsomal fractions prepared from cultured Cos-A2 cells transfected with human COX-1 and COX-2
Purified enzymes	Enzyme preparations from bovine or sheep seminal vesicles (COX-1) and sheep placenta (COX-2)
Recombinant enzymes	Human recombinant COX-1 and COX-2
	Murine recombinant COX-1 and COX-2

The longer the half-life, the smaller the fluctuation in the synovial fluid/plasma ratios which is illustrated by piroxicam with a ratio of 0.7 at maximal and minimal plasma and synovial concentrations. This difference in synovial fluid/plasma concentrations is an important factor in the variation of differential COX-2/COX-1 inhibition with time.

DIFFERENTIAL INHIBITION OF COX-1 AND COX-2

Experimental models to study differential COX-2/COX-1 inhibition by NSAIDs

A variety of cell lines expressing COX and purified or recombinant enzyme preparations have been introduced to study the effects of drugs on COX-1 and COX-2 (Table 2). The intrinsic activity of NSAIDs for COX-1 and COX-2 inhibition expressed as the IC_{50} varies between systems. Therefore, neither IC_{50} values themselves nor COX-2/COX-1 ratios of IC_{50} values from different systems can be directly compared (Table 3).

The results from these different test systems vary with changes in experimental conditions and assay procedures. This makes interpretation and comparison of the results difficult. The experimental conditions used in vitro should always try to reflect the pharmacokinetic parameters of the drug in vivo. Assay systems which resemble physiological conditions are the most appropriate for measurement of COX inhibition. Assay systems with intact cells appear to be more representative of the drug effects on target tissues than cell-free systems.

The influence of experimental conditions on dose–response curves for COX

Table 3   COX-2/COX-1 ratios from different test systems (IC_{50} values expressed in μmol/L)

	Guinea pig macrophages[14]			Human recombinant in Cos cells[15]			Human whole blood[16,17]		
	COX-2 IC_{50}	COX-1 IC_{50}	Ratio	COX-2 IC_{50}	COX-1 IC_{50}	Ratio	COX-2 IC_{50}	COX-1 IC_{50}	Ratio
Diclofenac	0.00191	0.000855	2.2	0.001	0.0026	0.39	–	–	–
Indomethacin	0.00636	0.00021	30	0.03	0.019	1.58	0.36	0.70	0.51
Ibuprofen	–	–	–	15.72	2.26	6.96	18.4	9.2	2
Naproxen	–	–	–	7.08	0.33	21.5	25.4	14.3	1.8
Meloxicam	0.00191	0.00577	0.33	0.16	2.24	0.07	0.43	4.8	0.09
Piroxicam	0.175	0.00527	33	0.98	2.03	0.48	–	–	–

inhibition has also been demonstrated by comparing COX inhibitory activity in intact Cos cells expressing human recombinant COX and in microsomal preparations from these cells. All agents were more potent in the intact system than in microsomal fractions[15]. These findings suggest that physicochemical factors affecting trans-membrane transport and intracellular trapping of the agent contribute to the magnitude and duration of COX inhibition at the intracellular target site.

NSAIDs have a very similar plasma protein binding and a 'free fraction' of approximately 1% of the total drug concentration is necessary for target tissue partitioning and trans-membrane transport. The amount of drug available as the 'free fraction' is influenced by differences in the protein content and nature of synovial fluid and pH, although this will affect all NSAIDs to a similar extent.

Some assays measuring NSAID activity in vitro are performed in the absence of proteins, however, the guinea-pig macrophage test[14], the Cos cell line expressing human COX-1 and COX-2[15], and the whole blood test using stimulated human monocytes[16] are conducted in the presence of protein and more accurately represent physiological or pathophysiological conditions in human disease.

NSAID inhibitory activity against COX-1 and COX-2

The COX-2/COX-1 ratios obtained for a range of NSAIDs in three different test systems are illustrated in Table 3. As discussed in the previous section there is considerable variation between test systems, and the COX-2/COX-1 ratios of IC_{50} values cannot be compared across the systems. In the guinea pig macrophage test system[14], indomethacin and piroxicam were more potent against COX-1 than COX-2, diclofenac was approximately equipotent against the two isoforms and meloxicam was more potent against COX-2 than COX-1. In Cos cells expressing human recombinant COX[15], naproxen and ibuprofen were more potent against COX-1 than COX-2, while diclofenac, indomethacin and piroxicam were approximately equipotent against both isoforms. Meloxicam, in contrast, was more potent against COX-2 than COX-1, suggesting selectivity towards COX-2.

By comparing the COX-2/COX-1 ratio calculated from the IC_{50} for both enzymes in different cell lines the NSAIDs can be ranked with respect to selectivity towards COX-2 or COX-1. A comparison of COX inhibition dose–response curves has shown preferential inhibition of COX-1 over COX-2 by indomethacin, ibuprofen, piroxicam and naproxen, equipotent COX-2/COX-1 inhibitory activity for diclofenac, and preferential inhibition of COX-2 over COX-1 for meloxicam[14,15].

DEFINITION OF RISK/BENEFIT INDEX

The relationship between drug concentration, time and COX inhibitory effects defines the pharmacological and therapeutic profile of the drug and reflects the time course and magnitude of differential COX-2/COX-1 inhibition. By combining pharmacokinetic and pharmacodynamic ratios in relation to drug levels at different times, it is possible to define a pharmacological drug profile (risk/benefit index).

Pharmacokinetic profiles are defined by the drug concentration/time course in the systemic circulation and the synovial system. This reflects the site, rate and extent of absorption following oral administration, distribution into and persistence in the target compartments for efficacy and toxicity, and mechanism and route of excretion.

Pharmacokinetic *ratios* express the synovial fluid/plasma concentration at a defined time point after drug administration.

Pharmacodynamic profiles are defined by the drug concentration/COX inhibitory effect relationship in vitro, in animal models or in patients.

Pharmacodynamic *ratios* express the differential inhibitory activity for both COX isoforms at the experimental conditions of assay and do not reflect the time course of inhibition.

A risk/benefit index has been derived from pharmacokinetic and pharmacodynamic parameters by constructing time/drug concentration/COX inhibitory profiles. Differences in kinetic and dynamic ratios of the NSAIDs translate into major differences in the risk/benefit index and are related to their clinical efficacy and toxicity.

The risk/benefit index has been calculated at mean and maximum plasma concentrations after drug administration ($C_{mean\ plasma}$ and $C_{max\ plasma}$)

- from the pharmacodynamic ratio (COX-2/COX-1 inhibition), and
- the pharmacokinetic ratio (synovial fluid/systemic drug concentration).

The relative COX inhibitory activity at the corresponding synovial fluid/plasma concentrations can be quantified by this index.

$$\text{Risk/benefit index} = \frac{IC_{50}\ COX\text{-}2/IC_{50}\ COX\text{-}1}{[\text{synovial fluid}]\ [\text{plasma}]}$$

Agents with a high synovial fluid/plasma concentration ratio and a low COX-2/COX-1 ratio have a low risk/benefit index and vice versa. It is evident that this index calculation results in a larger difference between the NSAIDs compared with the COX-2/COX-1 ratio.

- *COX-2/COX-1 ratio:* between 21.5 (naproxen) and 0.07 (meloxicam)
- *Risk/benefit index:* between 59.7 (naproxen) and 0.13 (meloxicam) at $C_{max\ plasma}$

RISK/BENEFIT INDEX OF STANDARD NSAIDs

The risk/benefit index was calculated using published data on pharmacokinetics and COX-2/COX-1 ratios generated by intact cells with recombinant human COX[15]. Indices were calculated at $C_{max\,plasma}$ and $C_{mean\,plasma}$ and are presented in Table 4 for a range of NSAIDs.

The indices attributed to individual agents present evidence for marked differences not only between NSAIDs, but also at different time points during standard dosing intervals of individual NSAIDs. In particular, NSAIDs with a short half-life will have fluctuating plasma and synovial concentrations during a dosing interval. The synovial fluid/plasma concentration ratio for diclofenac, indomethacin and ibuprofen is low between 30 min and 3 hours after dosing, representing a high systemic level relative to the synovial fluid concentration. However, with increasing time there is a shift towards a higher synovial concentration and, therefore, an increase in the synovial fluid/plasma concentration ratio. Although the pharmacokinetic profile is similar for diclofenac, ibuprofen and indomethacin, there are major differences in differential COX-2/COX-1 inhibitory activity. Diclofenac has been shown to be equipotent against COX-1 and COX-2 while ibuprofen and indomethacin are more selective against COX-1 than COX-2 (Table 3). The risk/benefit index calculated at $C_{max\,plasma}$ reflects these differences. Diclofenac has a risk/benefit index of 1.1 compared with 12.2 for indomethacin and 13.9 for ibuprofen.

NSAIDs with a longer half-life show smaller fluctuations in their synovial fluid/plasma concentration ratio with time of dosing and at steady state the ratios are constant. Following once daily administration of 20 mg piroxicam, steady state plasma concentrations are established after 3 weeks and the synovial fluid/plasma ratio is approximately 0.7, this correlates with a risk/benefit index of 0.7 at C_{max} and C_{mean} (Table 4).

Naproxen steady-state plasma concentrations were established after administration of 500 mg bid naproxen daily and under these conditions a synovial fluid/plasma concentration ratio of 0.36 at C_{max} and 0.66 at C_{mean} was achieved. The risk/benefit indices calculated from these ratios are 59.7 at C_{max} and 32.6 at C_{mean}.

Recent studies conducted with meloxicam (one week of administration of 15 mg or 7.5 mg daily) have allowed the calculation at steady-state plasma concentrations of the synovial fluid/plasma concentration ratio (0.53 at C_{max} and 0.48 at C_{mean}). This corresponds to a risk/benefit index of 0.13 at C_{max} and 0.15 at C_{mean}.

The risk/benefit index (calculated at C_{max}) of the NSAIDs under comparison covers a wide range with naproxen (59.7), ibuprofen (13.9) and indomethacin (12.2) at one end of the spectrum and meloxicam (0.13) at the other end.

CLINICAL SAFETY PROFILES OF NSAIDs

Clinical data on the frequency of severe gastrointestinal adverse events associated with NSAID use would appear to be consistent with the ranking of NSAIDs according to the risk/benefit index. A global analysis of clinical trials with naproxen (750–1000 mg/day), diclofenac (100 mg CR/day), piroxicam (20 mg/day), and

Table 4   *IC$_{50}$ values, COX-2/COX-1 ratios, synovial fluid/plasma ratios, and risk/benefit index of various NSAIDs*

	IC_{50} COX-2	IC_{50} COX-1	COX-2/COX-1 ratio	C_{SF}/C_P at $C_{max\,P}$	C_{SF}/C_P at $C_{mean\,P}$	Risk/benefit index at $C_{max\,P}$	Risk/benefit index at $C_{mean\,P}$
Diclofenac 50 mg	0.32 ng/ml	0.83 ng/ml	0.39	0.35	–	1.1	–
100 mg CR				–	0.8	–	0.49
Indomethacin 50 mg	10.7 ng/ml	6.8 ng/ml	1.58	0.13	–	12.2	–
Ibuprofen 600 mg repeated doses (day 3)	3.24 μg/ml	0.47 μg/ml	6.96	0.5	–	13.9	–
Naproxen 500 mg bid (steady state)	1.63 μg/ml	0.076 μg/ml	21.5	0.36	0.66	59.7	32.6
Meloxicam 15 mg (steady state)	0.056 μg/ml	0.79 μg/ml	0.07	0.53	0.48	0.13	0.15
Piroxicam 20 mg (steady state)	0.33 μg/ml	0.67 μg/ml	0.48	0.7	0.7	0.7	0.7

COX data from Churchill et al. 1996[15]

SF = synovial fluid; P = plasma

meloxicam (7.5 mg/day and 15 mg/day), reported that the incidence of severe GI adverse events (meloxicam 7.5 mg: 1.7%; meloxicam 15 mg; 1.7%; piroxicam: 4.9%; diclofenac; 4.9%; naproxen: 7.8%; $p < 0.05$) and life-threatening GI adverse events (meloxicam 7.5 mg: 0.1%; meloxicam 15 mg: 0.2%; piroxicam: 1.2%; diclofenac: 0.6%; naproxen: 2.1%; $p < 0.05$) was significantly less in meloxicam treated patients compared with the other treatment groups[18]. Furthermore, in a study which used endoscopic assessments to investigate the toxic effects of NSAIDs on the gut using the Lanza scoring system[19], a surprisingly high frequency of clinically significant mucosal lesions in the stomach and the duodenum were shown to be associated with chronic use of diclofenac, piroxicam, indomethacin, naproxen and ibuprofen[20]. Ibuprofen was associated with a higher frequency of lesions than the comparators, and diclofenac caused less GI damage than the other agents (Table 5).

In contrast, ibuprofen has been shown to have low toxicity on the gut in observational and epidemiological studies. In the European observational study SPALA (Safety Profile of Anti-rheumatics in Long-term Administration)[21] ibuprofen had the lowest frequency of GI adverse events (Table 5), although this may be related to the low mean daily dose in this study which was less than half that usually recognised as anti-inflammatory. That ibuprofen is often prescribed at lower doses than those used for anti-inflammatory activity may also explain the findings from four recent epidemiological studies performed in the UK, Australia and New Zealand[22–25], ibuprofen has a low toxicity on the gut, whereas piroxicam has a high toxicity. Such studies reflect only a small segment of toxicity on the gut seen in clinical practice.

There is an ongoing debate regarding the clinical relevance of in vitro data and whether ratios defining COX-2 inhibition relative to COX-1 inhibition represent an indication of likely gut toxicity. The rank order of COX-2/COX-1 ratios in vitro using intact cells expressing human recombinant COX (Table 4) generally correlates with rank orders for risk/benefit indices (Table 4) and is consistent with the clinical trial evidence for gut toxicity. That this ranking is not consistent with the results of epidemiological studies (Table 5) remains to be elucidated; however, it may reflect the prescription pattern for drugs such as ibuprofen which is commonly used in low (analgesic) doses rather than anti-inflammatory doses. On the other hand, the lack of dose flexibility in practice for piroxicam may result in a higher incidence of GI side effects; this may particularly affect at-risk patients.

Summary

The various members of the NSAID class exhibit differing selectivity towards COX-1 and COX-2 and this has been investigated in a number of in vitro systems. The tissue distribution of activity (relevant to arthritis) is different for the two isoforms of the COX enzyme and while COX-2 activity is expressed in synovial cells, COX-1 activity is expressed in thrombocytes, the gastrointestinal mucosa, and the kidney. A risk/benefit index has been defined which combines information on the differential COX-2/COX-1 inhibition with a quantitative measure of the relative NSAID distribution between the synovial fluid and plasma. The risk/benefit index has been calculated for a number of standard NSAIDs and covers a range between >20 and

Table 5 *GI toxicity of NSAIDs from epidemiological and endoscopy studies*

	1	2	3	4	5
Endoscopic studies					
Geis[20] – study	diclofenac	piroxicam	indomethacin	naproxen	ibuprofen
number of patients	461	226	180	247	173
% with GI lesions	29.3	31.4	32.2	35.2	37
Observational study					
18 400 patients (SPALA)[21]	ibuprofen	diclofenac	piroxicam	naproxen	indomethacin
daily dose	>1200 mg/day	100 mg/day	20 mg/day	>750 mg/day	100 mg/day
number of patients	2080	8251	880	541	1855
% with GI adverse events	10	10.9	11.1	12.4	13.4
Epidemiological studies					
Langman[22] – study UK	ibuprofen	diclofenac	naproxen	indomethacin	piroxicam
Relative risk	2	4.2	9.1	11.3	13.7
Rodriguez[23] – study UK	ibuprofen	naproxen	diclofenac	indomethacin	piroxicam
Relative risk	2.9	3.1	3.9	6.3	18
Henry[24] – study AUS	ibuprofen	diclofenac	indomethacin	naproxen	piroxicam
Relative risk	0.7	1.7	2.5	2.8	4.8
Savage[25] – study NZ	ibuprofen	diclofenac	naproxen	piroxicam	indomethacin
Relative risk	1.9	3.3	5.1	6.4	13.9

<0.5. NSAIDs such as naproxen, indomethacin and ibuprofen are at one end of the spectrum with risk/benefit indices greater than 10, whereas meloxicam is at the other end with a risk/benefit index of 0.13.

Classification of the NSAIDs has historically been based on their structure. However, with the recent discovery of two isoforms of the COX enzyme and the differences in selectivity towards COX-1 and COX-2 demonstrated by most of the currently available NSAIDs, a new method of classification would appear timely. The risk/benefit index by combining both pharmacodynamic and pharmacokinetic variables accounts for both the relative distribution of the NSAID into the COX-1 or COX-2 expressing compartments and the relative selectivity towards the COX isoforms.

References

1. Gottlieb NL. The art and science of non-steroidal anti-inflammatory drug selection. Semin Arthritis. 1985;15(suppl 2):1.
2. Furst DE. Are there differences among nonsteroidal antiinflammatory drugs? Arthritis Rheum. 1994;37:1–9.
3. Day RO, Graham GG, Williams KM, Brooks PM. Variability in response to NSAIDs: Fact or fiction? Drugs. 1988;36:643–51.
4. Brooks PM, Day RO. Nonsteroidal antiinflammatory drugs – differences and similarities. N Engl J Med. 1991;324:1716–25.
5. Engelhardt G, Homma D, Schlegel K, Utzmann R, Schnitzler C. Anti-inflammatory, analgesic, antipyretic and related properties of mcloxicam, a new non-steroidal anti-inflammatory agent with favourable gastrointestinal tolerance. Inflamm Res. 1995;44:423–33.
6. Wiesenberg-Boettcher I, Schweizer A, Green JR, Mueller K, Maerki F, Pfeilschifter J. The pharmacological profile of CGP 28238, a novel highly potent anti-inflammatory compound. Drugs Exp Clin Res. 1989;15;501–9.
7. Fowler PD, Shadforth MF, Crook PR, John VA. Plasma and synovial fluid concentrations of diclofenac sodium and its major hydroxylated metabolites during long-term treatment of rheumatoid arthritis. Eur J Clin Pharmacol. 1983;25:389–94.
8. Fowler PD, Dawes PT, John VA, Shotton PA. Plasma and synovial fluid concentrations of diclofenac sodium and its hydroxylated metabolites during once-daily administration of a 100 mg slow-release formulation. Eur J Clin Pharmacol. 1986;31:469–72.
9. Emori WE, Champion GD, Bluestone R, Paulus HE. Simultaneous pharmacokinetics of indomethacin in serum and synovial fluid. Ann Rheum Dis. 1983;32:433–5.
10. Gallo JM, Gall EP, Gillespie WR, Albert KS, Perrier D. Ibuprofen kinetics in plasma and synovial fluid of arthritic patients. J Clin Pharmacol. 1986;26:65–70.
11. Day RO, Francis H, Vial J, Geisslinger G, Williams KM. Naproxen concentrations in plasma and synovial fluid and effects on prostanoid concentrations. J Rheumatol. 1995;22:2295–303.
12. Degner F, Heinzel G, Busch U. Transsynovial kinetics of meloxicam. Scand J Rheumatol. 1995; 98(suppl 98):121.
13. Kurowski M, Dunky A. Transsynovial kinetics of piroxicam in patients with rheumatoid arthritis. Eur J Clin Pharmacol. 1988;34:401–6.
14. Engelhardt G, Bögel R, Schnitzler C, Utzmann R. Meloxicam: Influence on arachidonic acid metabolism. In vitro findings – Part I. Biochem Pharmacol. 1996;51:21–8.
15. Churchill L, Graham AG, Shih C-K, Pauletti D, Farina PR, Grob PM. Selective inhibition of human cyclo-oxygenase-2 by meloxicam. Inflammopharmacology. 1996;4:125–35.
16. Patrignani P, Panara MR, Greco A et al. Biochemical and pharmacological characterization of the cyclooxygenase activity of human blood prostaglandin endoperoxide synthases. J Pharmacol Exp Ther. 1994;271:1705–12.
17. Pairet M, Engelhardt G. Differential inhibition of COX-1 and COX-2 *in vitro* and pharmacological profile *in vivo* of NSAIDs. In: Vane J, Botting J, Botting R (eds): Improved Non-steroid

Anti-inflammatory Drugs – COX-2 Enzyme Inhibitors. Dordrecht/Boston/London: Kluwer Academic Publishers; 1996;103–19.

18. Distel M, Mueller C, Bluhmki E, Fries J. Safety of meloxicam: A global analysis of clinical trials. Br J Rheumatol. 1996;35(1):68–77.

19. Lanza FL. Gastrointestinal toxicity of new NSAIDs. Am J Gastroenterol. 1993;88:1318–23.

20. Geis GS, Stead H, Wallemark CB, Nicholson PA. Prevalence of mucosal lesions in the stomach and duodenum due to chronic use of NSAID in patients with rheumatoid arthritis or osteoarthritis, an interim report on prevention by misoprostol of diclofenac associated lesions. J Rheumatol Suppl. 1991;28:11–14.

21. A report from the SPALA Project. The Design of SPALA (Safety Profile of Antirheumatics in Long-term Administration): an intensive monitoring system for NSAIDs. Eur J Clin Pharmacol. 1988;34:529–30.

22. Langman MJS. Anti-inflammatory drugs and the gut: ulcerative damage and protection from cancer. Proceedings of Symposium: New Insights into Anti-inflammatory Therapy and its Benefits, Cannes, October 1994. Macclesfield, UK: Adelphi Communications Ltd.

23. Garcia Rodriguez LA, Jick H. Risk of upper gastrointestinal bleeding and perforation associated with individual non-steroidal anti-inflammatory drugs. Lancet. 1994;343:769–72.

24. Henry D, Dobson A, Turner C. Variability in the risk of major gastrointestinal complications from non aspirin non steroidal anti-inflammatory drugs. Gastroenterology. 1993;105:1978–88.

25. Savage RL, Moller PW, Ballantyne CL, Wells JE. Variation in the risk of peptic ulcer complications with non steroidal anti-inflammatory drug therapy. Arthritis Rheum. 1993;36:84–90.

12 Clinical experience with meloxicam, a selective COX-2 inhibitor

W. BOLTEN

Gastrointestinal side effects caused by inhibition of cytoprotective prostaglandins in the gastric mucosa are a major drawback to the use of non-steroid anti-inflammatory drugs (NSAIDs) in the treatment of rheumatic disease. The recent discovery of two isoforms of the cyclooxygenase (COX) enzyme may provide a way forward in NSAID development, allowing for sustained efficacy with improved tolerability. The constitutive isoform, COX-1, maintains physiological prostaglandin production and its inhibition causes the characteristic side effects of NSAIDs such as gastrointestinal and renal toxicity. By contrast, inhibition of the inducible inflammatory isoform, COX-2, is responsible for the undoubted therapeutic efficacy of NSAIDs. NSAIDs that have a higher activity against COX-2 than against COX-1 may therefore have fewer side effects, while maintaining efficacy. Many of the currently available NSAIDs are selective for COX-1 or are equipotent against both COX-1 and COX-2. NSAIDs such as meloxicam, which are more selective for COX-2 than for COX-1, have been developed and are efficacious in the treatment of rheumatic disease. Drugs which are highly selective for COX-2 are presently being developed and studied.

Epidemiological studies with existing NSAIDs suggest that there is a relationship between high selectivity for COX-1 and a poorer gastrointestinal safety profile. However, only limited clinical results are available with the newer, more selective or highly selective COX-2 inhibitors in order to allow a judgement on the impact of these drugs on arthritis therapy.

The need for safer NSAIDs can be appreciated when the characteristics of the patient population are considered. Elderly patients are the largest users of NSAIDs due to their increased risk of conditions such as osteoarthritis. It has been estimated that about 15% of the UK population aged 60 and over are taking non-aspirin NSAIDs at any one time and about the same proportion are taking aspirin alone or concomitantly with other NSAIDs. Moreover, the number of elderly patients using these drugs will rise as the ageing population increases. The age of the patient is one of the major risk factors for gastrointestinal complications associated with NSAID therapy. Age-related changes in gastroduodenal physiology mean that gastrointestinal injuries caused by NSAIDs are less likely to heal in the elderly. It also appears that elderly patients are less likely to experience any warning symptoms of such damage and are most likely to die of gastrointestinal complications.

Physicians need to be able to provide effective pain relief to patients with osteo-arthritis and rheumatoid arthritis and, while this is available with current NSAIDs, it is accompanied by a serious concern about side effects. The development of selective COX-2 inhibitors which could provide sustained efficacy with a lower incidence of gastrointestinal and renal toxicity would provide the physician with a more acceptable treatment. One new, more selective COX-2 inhibitor for which clinical results are available is meloxicam. This review will examine the potential role of selective COX-2 inhibitors in the treatment of osteoarthritis and rheumatoid arthritis by presenting the clinical data obtained with meloxicam.

PHARMACOKINETICS

The pharmacokinetic profile of meloxicam is essentially linear and it is characterized by almost complete absorption over a prolonged phase. Steady-state conditions are achieved in approximately 3–5 days: faster than seen with other NSAIDs such as piroxicam (7–12 days) and tenoxicam (9–14 days)[1]. The half-life of meloxicam is approximately 20h, which supports the recommendation of once-daily dosing whilst reducing the risk of any drug accumulation. Meloxicam is extensively metabolized in the liver; all the metabolites are inactive and therefore do not contribute to the action of the parent compound. Meloxicam undergoes balanced excretion, approximately 50% being excreted via the kidneys and 50% in the faeces.

It is important to investigate any potential changes in the pharmacokinetic profile of a drug (and consequently the requirement for dosage adjustments) when it is administered to special patient populations, such as the elderly or those with renal or hepatic impairment. The high plasma protein binding of meloxicam (>99%) may influence the pharmacokinetic profile in special patient populations. No dosage adjustments were found to be necessary in elderly patients (more than 65 years old), patients with liver insufficiency associated with liver cirrhosis or patients with mild (creatinine clearance of 41–60 ml/min) or moderate (creatinine clearance of 20–40 ml/min) renal impairment[1]. Only minor dosage adjustments were required even in patients with end-stage renal failure.

NSAID treatment for rheumatoid arthritis or osteoarthritis is often chronic and patients may require drug therapy for other clinical conditions at the same time. Concomitant administration of meloxicam with other drugs including digoxin, cimetidine, antacids, furosemide, warfarin and methotrexate did not result in any clinically significant interactions[1].

STUDIES IN HEALTHY VOLUNTEERS

Urinary excretion of PGE$_2$ after treatment with meloxicam and indomethacin

In vitro and animal studies have confirmed that meloxicam more selectively inhibits COX-2 relative to COX-1. In a randomized cross-over study in 12 healthy volunteers, meloxicam (7.5 mg once daily) and indomethacin (25 mg three times daily) were compared in terms of their effects on platelet aggregation and urinary excretion of prostaglandin E_2 (PGE_2) (a measure of renal safety), both of which are COX-1 dependent.

Maximal platelet aggregation was significantly inhibited by indomethacin compared with pretreatment values (11% vs. 82%; $p < 0.001$); meloxicam had no effect on platelet aggregation compared with pretreatment values (80% vs. 82%). Similarly, urinary PGE_2 excretion was significantly reduced by indomethacin compared with pretreatment levels (24 vs. 47 nmol/mol creatinine; $p < 0.05$); again meloxicam had no effect on this parameter (43 vs. 47 nmol/mol creatinine).

Meloxicam, therefore, was COX-1 sparing at a dose which is clinically as effective as the established NSAIDs diclofenac (100 mg) and piroxicam (20 mg).

Mean total endoscopic scores

Gastrointestinal damage due to NSAIDs can be a significant problem. Since meloxicam selectively inhibits COX-2, however, it should result in less gastrointestinal toxicity than other NSAIDs. This has been confirmed in animal studies and a recent study has investigated the gastrointestinal toxicity in healthy volunteers[2].

Endoscopic methods were used to assess the gastrointestinal safety of meloxicam in a double-blind, randomized, parallel-group study of 51 healthy male volunteers who received placebo, piroxicam 20 mg/day, meloxicam 7.5 mg/day or meloxicam 15 mg/day for 28 days[2]. Endoscopic scores showed a significant ($p < 0.05$) difference between piroxicam compared with meloxicam 7.5 mg and placebo at the end of the study. There was a significantly ($p < 0.001$) higher number of withdrawals due to poor endoscopic score in the piroxicam group compared with the other groups. Upper gastrointestinal ulcers occurred in six subjects given piroxicam (all of whom were withdrawn from the study); no ulcers were seen in the placebo or meloxicam 7.5 mg groups while one patient in the meloxicam 15 mg group developed a gastric ulcer but was not withdrawn prematurely.

The improved gastrointestinal safety of meloxicam over that of piroxicam 20 mg/day was therefore confirmed in this small study in healthy volunteers.

EFFICACY

Data from a total of 4175 patients (1820 of whom had osteoarthritis and 1889 of whom had rheumatoid arthritis) are included in the meloxicam database (Table 1). These patients had been treated with meloxicam doses of 7.5 mg or 15 mg for mean periods of 70 and 128 days respectively. The clinical data appertaining to those patients with osteoarthritis and rheumatoid arthritis will be discussed below.

Osteoarthritis

Placebo-controlled study

Meloxicam at doses of 7.5 mg and 15 mg has been shown to be significantly more effective than placebo in patients with osteoarthritis[3]. A double blind, 3-week,

Table 1   The meloxicam patient database: an overview

	Meloxicam 7.5 mg	Meloxicam 15 mg
Total	893	3282
Rheumatoid arthritis	572	1317
Osteoarthritis	309	1511
Other indications	0	298
Exposure		
Mean (days)	70	128
Median (days)	22	29
Mean age (years)	59	57
Elderly (>65 years)	33%	33%
Sex		
Male	265	1176
Female	628	2106

randomized, placebo-controlled study was carried out in 41 European centres and compared meloxicam 7.5 mg/day ($n=140$) and 15 mg/day ($n=134$) with placebo ($n=137$) in patients with osteoarthritis of the knee. After 3 weeks of treatment, meloxicam 7.5 mg and 15 mg were significantly ($p<0.05$) more effective than placebo in terms of mean reduction in pain on movement as measured on a 100 mm visual analogue scale (VAS). The 15 mg dose was also significantly ($p<0.05$) more effective than placebo in terms of mean reduction in pain at rest and the mean global efficacy score.

Comparative studies with other NSAIDs

Four major double-blind, comparative studies have compared the efficacy of meloxicam (7.5 mg and 15 mg) with that of piroxicam (20 mg) and diclofenac (100 mg SR), in patients with osteoarthritis of the hip or knee. Meloxicam (15 mg) has been compared with piroxicam (20 mg) in both a short-term (6-week)[4] and a longer-term (6-month) study[5]. In the short-term study, meloxicam 15 mg/day ($n=129$) and piroxicam 20 mg/day ($n=127$) were administered to patients with osteoarthritis of the hip, and an assessment of pain and global efficacy was recorded by the patient using a 100 mm VAS[4]. Both meloxicam and piroxicam showed a continuous reduction in pain on movement during the study and there was a trend in favour of meloxicam in all the secondary efficacy parameters: reduction in pain at rest, reduction in index of severity from baseline to final observation and global efficacy. However, none of the differences achieved statistical significance.

The long-term efficacy of meloxicam 15 mg/day ($n=306$) and piroxicam 20 mg/day ($n=149$) was evaluated in a double-blind, 6-month, randomized, parallel-group study in patients with osteoarthritis of the hip or knee[5]. Patients in both treatment groups had marked reductions in overall pain, as measured on a 100 mm VAS. After 6 months' treatment, the mean reduction from baseline was 31 mm with meloxicam and 27 mm with piroxicam (Figure 1). Meloxicam and piroxicam

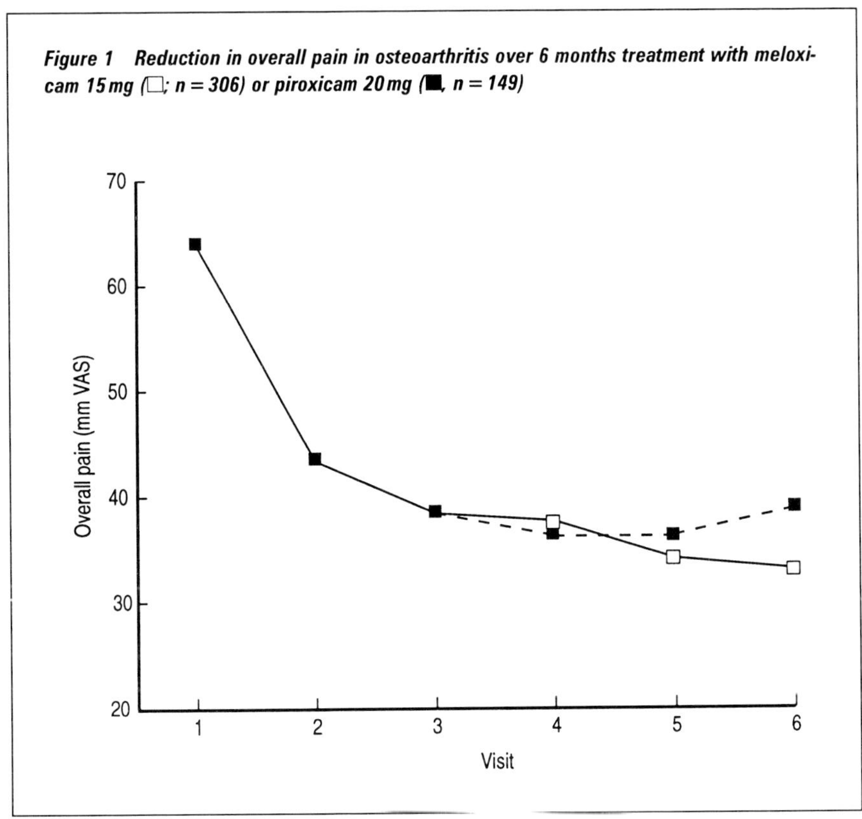

Figure 1   Reduction in overall pain in osteoarthritis over 6 months treatment with meloxicam 15 mg (□; n = 306) or piroxicam 20 mg (■, n = 149)

produced similar improvements in pain on movement, duration of stiffness after rest and quality of life. The global efficacy score at the end of treatment was also similar in both groups.

Meloxicam has also been compared with the well established and widely used NSAID diclofenac in a short-term (6-week) and a longer-term (6-month) study. The short-term study was carried out in 23 European centres and compared meloxicam 15 mg/day ($n=128$) and diclofenac SR 100 mg/day ($n=130$) in patients with osteoarthritis of the knee[6]. A relatively large reduction in pain on movement occurred after 7 days of treatment in both groups, as measured on a 100 mm VAS. This was followed by a gradual, but less pronounced, reduction over the remainder of the study in both groups; the mean improvement from day 21 to the end of the study was more pronounced in the meloxicam group. Meloxicam and diclofenac were equally effective in terms of reducing pain at rest and improvement in the total index of severity. There was a trend in favour of meloxicam in terms of global efficacy and paracetamol consumption. These differences were not statistically significant.

The long-term, comparative study was carried out in 52 general practitioner centres in the UK and compared meloxicam 7.5 mg/day ($n=169$) and diclofenac SR

100 mg/day ($n = 167$) in patients with osteoarthritis of the hip or knee[7]. Both meloxicam and diclofenac resulted in a similar marked reduction in overall pain and pain on movement. The maximum reduction in both parameters was achieved after 1 month in both groups. The median dose of paracetamol required during the study was significantly lower in the meloxicam group than in the diclofenac group (185 vs. 245 mg/day; $p < 0.05$). There was also a trend in favour of meloxicam for a greater amelioration in duration of stiffness after rest at the end of the study. Meloxicam and diclofenac were equally effective in terms of global efficacy and improvement in quality of life.

In conclusion, five large double-blind, placebo-controlled or comparative studies have demonstrated the efficacy of meloxicam in the treatment of osteoarthritis. Meloxicam in the dose range 7.5–15 mg/day has been shown to be equally as effective as the standard therapies, piroxicam 20 mg and diclofenac 100 mg SR.

Rheumatoid arthritis

Placebo-controlled study

A double-blind, 3-week, randomized, placebo-controlled study was carried out in patients with rheumatoid arthritis (at least 6 months' duration; American College of Rheumatology (ACR) functional class of I, II or III; requirement for NSAIDs for at least 6 months continuously prior to study) in order to compare meloxicam 7.5 mg/day ($n = 159$) and 15 mg/day ($n = 162$) with placebo ($n = 147$)[8]. After 3 weeks of treatment, meloxicam 7.5 mg and 15 mg were significantly ($p < 0.05$) superior to placebo in reducing disease activity as assessed by the patient, whilst meloxicam 15 mg was significantly ($p < 0.05$) superior to placebo in reducing disease activity as assessed by both the patient and the investigator. Both doses of meloxicam were also significantly ($p < 0.05$) better than placebo in reducing the number of painful/tender joints. Significantly ($p < 0.001$) more patients in the placebo group discontinued therapy due to lack of efficacy (16%) compared with the 7.5 mg and 15 mg meloxicam groups (4% and 4%). Global efficacy of meloxicam 15 mg was significantly ($p < 0.01$) better than placebo and meloxicam 7.5 mg, while meloxicam 7.5 mg was significantly ($p < 0.05$) better than placebo. Both doses of meloxicam were also significantly ($p < 0.05$) superior to placebo with respect to the mean score for activities of daily living and the number of patients requiring concomitant paracetamol.

Comparative studies with other NSAIDs

Two major double-blind, multicentre studies have compared the efficacy of meloxicam with the standard NSAIDs, piroxicam and naproxen, in patients with rheumatoid arthritis.

The short-term efficacy of meloxicam (15 mg/day) was compared with piroxicam (20 mg/day) in a double-blind, 3-week, multicentre, randomized study in 276 patients (141 meloxicam, 135 piroxicam) with rheumatoid arthritis (Steinbrocker progression scale of I, II or III and a Steinbrocker functional scale of II or III)[9]. Meloxicam and

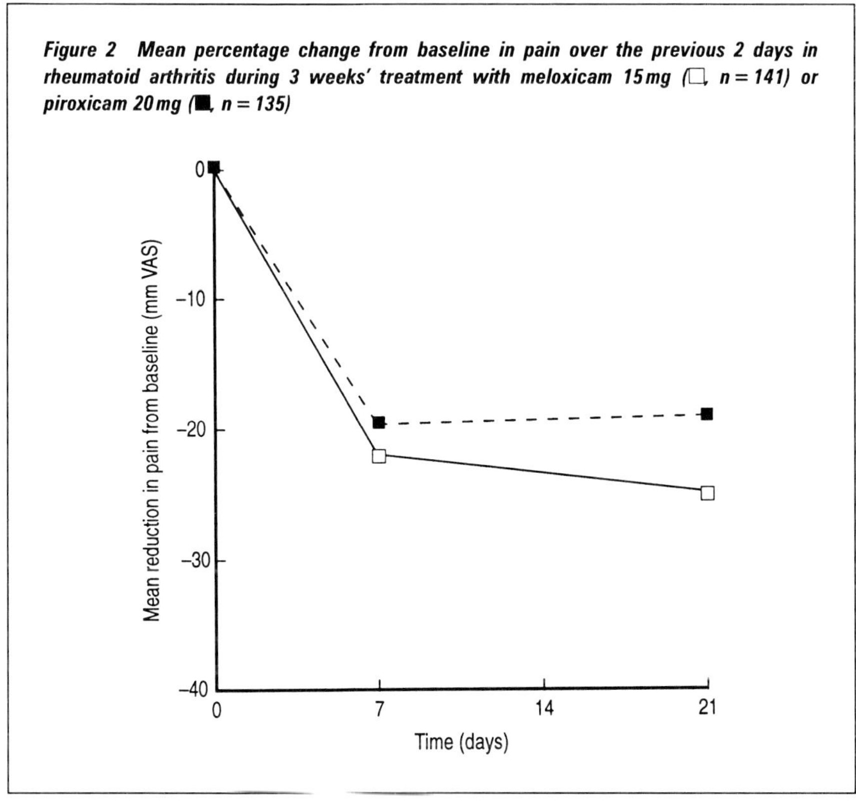

Figure 2 Mean percentage change from baseline in pain over the previous 2 days in rheumatoid arthritis during 3 weeks' treatment with meloxicam 15 mg (□, n = 141) or piroxicam 20 mg (■, n = 135)

piroxicam were equally effective, as assessed by global efficacy (patient and physician), mean percentage reduction from baseline in pain on movement, pain at night and pain in the morning, the Ritchie joint index, the duration of morning stiffness and mean percentage reduction in pain over the previous 2 days (Figure 2). The number of withdrawals due to inadequate efficacy (meloxicam seven, piroxicam five) was also similar in both groups.

The long-term efficacy of meloxicam 7.5 mg/day ($n = 199$) in the treatment of rheumatoid arthritis has been compared with the established NSAID naproxen 750 mg/day ($n = 180$) in a double-blind, 6-month, randomized, multicentre, parallel-group study[10]. Patient and investigator assessments of global efficacy, measured on a VAS, were similar although naproxen was rated as slightly better. Both treatment groups showed significant ($p < 0.05$) improvements in grip strength and reductions in the number of painful/tender joints, the number of swollen joints, morning stiffness, pain at night, pain in the morning and difficulties with activities of daily living; there were no significant differences between the groups. Only swollen joint severity index was improved to a significantly ($p < 0.01$) greater extent with naproxen than with meloxicam. Erythrocyte sedimentation rate improved significantly with meloxicam

Table 2   Patient numbers in global safety analysis

	Total	OA or RA patients in double-blind studies only
Meloxicam 7.5 mg	893	881
Meloxicam 15 mg	3282	1590
Piroxicam 20 mg	906	689
Diclofenac 100 mg SR	324	324
Naproxen 750–1000 mg	243	243
Total	5648	3727

but not with naproxen. A significantly ($p < 0.05$) larger percentage of patients discontinued due to lack of efficacy in the meloxicam group (23.6%) compared with the naproxen group (14.4%).

In conclusion, three major double-blind, comparative studies have been conducted in more than 1100 patients with rheumatoid arthritis. Meloxicam in the dose range 7.5–15 mg/day was significantly more effective than placebo and at the dose of 15 mg was as effective as piroxicam 20 mg. Meloxicam 7.5 mg was as effective as naproxen 750 mg.

GLOBAL SAFETY ANALYSIS

A total of 5648 patients have been included in the global safety analysis of meloxicam (7.5 mg and 15 mg), piroxicam (20 mg), diclofenac (100 mg SR), and naproxen (750–1000 mg) (Table 2)[11]. This represents a broad database of clinical experience. The majority were suffering from osteoarthritis or rheumatoid arthritis and had been enrolled in double-blind, controlled studies (Table 2). Overall safety data were determined for the total population. However, sub-categories of gastrointestinal side effects were assessed only in osteoarthritis and rheumatoid arthritis patients enrolled in double-blind studies; this subpopulation is clearly the best controlled and most reliable.

Overview of side effects in global safety analysis

Table 3 lists side effects in different organ classes for the total safety population. Naproxen and diclofenac were associated with the highest incidence of side effects (60.5% and 56.2%, respectively) while the incidence was lowest with meloxicam 7.5 mg (43.0%), followed by piroxicam (43.8%) and meloxicam 15 mg (45.2%)[11]. Naproxen was associated with a very high incidence of gastrointestinal side effects (36.6%). The lowest incidence of gastrointestinal side effects was seen with meloxicam 7.5 mg (16.8%) and meloxicam 15 mg (18.3%). The only other side effect which occurred in more than 10% of patients was increased GOT (glutamate oxalate transaminase)/GPT (glutamate pyruvate transaminase) which occurred in 16.1% of patients treated with diclofenac SR.

Table 3 Overview of side effects in global safety analysis

	Meloxicam 7.5 mg (n=893)	Meloxicam 15 mg (n=3282)	Piroxicam 20 mg (n=906)	Diclofenac SR 100 mg (n=324)	Naproxen 750–1000 mg (n=243)
Gastrointestinal	16.8	18.3	20.2	26.5	36.6
CNS	7.7	7.6	6.6	6.8	7.8
↑ GOT/GPT	5.9	7.4	6.3	16.1	9.5
Skin/appendages	6.5	6.2	4.4	4.0	8.2
Respiratory system	6.2	7.3	3.6	6.2	6.2
Urinary system	4.4	5.3	4.9	3.1	4.9
↑ creatinine/BUN	0.5	0.4	0.9	0.3	0.4
Total	43.0	45.2	43.8	56.2	60.5

GOT = glutamate oxalate transaminase; GPT = glutamate pyruvate transaminase; BUN = blood urea nitrogen.

Values are percentage of treated patients experiencing each side effect

Gastrointestinal side effects

Gastrointestinal side effects are a significant problem with NSAID treatment. Survival curves, describing the total occurrence of gastrointestinal side effects over time in double-blind studies of patients with osteoarthritis or rheumatoid arthritis, are illustrated in Figure 3. As can be seen, the risk of gastrointestinal side effects was significantly ($p < 0.05$) greater with naproxen, piroxicam and diclofenac than with either dose of meloxicam[11]. Similarly, when survival curves describing the occurrence of severe gastrointestinal side effects over time in double-blind studies of patients with osteoarthritis or rheumatoid arthritis were constructed, the risk of occurrence was found to be significantly ($p < 0.05$) greater with naproxen, diclofenac and piroxicam than with either dose of meloxicam[11]. The incidence of upper gastrointestinal side effects, including dyspepsia, eructation, nausea, vomiting, gastric ulcer, duodenal ulcer, haematemesis and melaena, was significantly higher ($p < 0.05$) with naproxen than with either dose of meloxicam, while the incidence with diclofenac was also significantly ($p < 0.05$) higher than with the 7.5 mg dose of meloxicam.

As might be expected from the previous results the incidence of discontinuation due to gastrointestinal side effects over time in double-blind studies of patients with osteoarthritis or rheumatoid arthritis was significantly ($p < 0.05$) higher with diclofenac and naproxen than with either dose of meloxicam. The incidence with piroxicam was significantly ($p < 0.05$) higher than with 15 mg meloxicam.

Dyspepsia/abdominal pain

Dyspepsia and abdominal pain are two of the most common gastrointestinal adverse events with NSAIDs. A good safety profile with respect to these events will therefore improve patient tolerability and compliance. Survival curves describing the incidence of dyspepsia over time in double blind studies of patients with osteoarthritis or

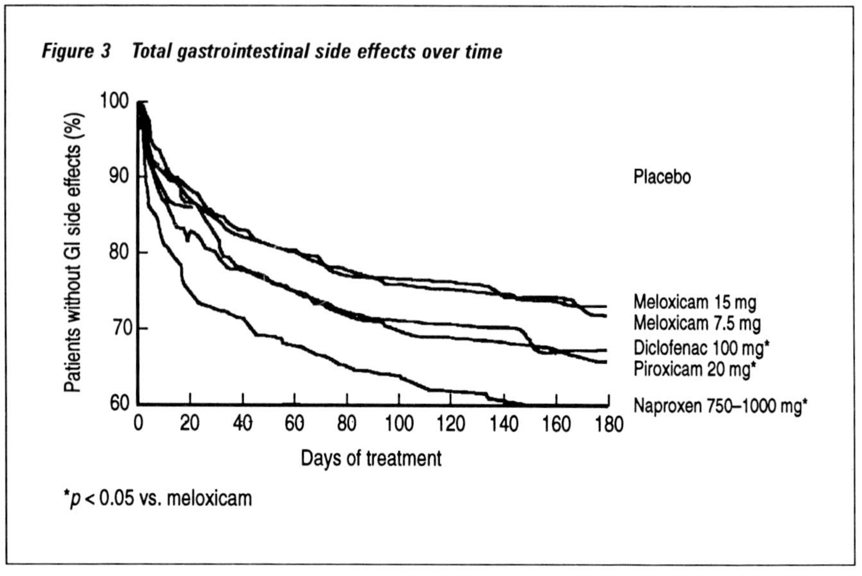

rheumatoid arthritis have shown that the risk is significantly ($p < 0.05$) greater with naproxen than with either dose of meloxicam. The risk with the 7.5 mg dose of meloxicam is also significantly ($p < 0.05$) less than with any of the other treatments. Similarly, survival curves describing the occurrence of abdominal pain over time have demonstrated that the risk is significantly ($p < 0.05$) greater with naproxen, piroxicam and diclofenac than with either dose of meloxicam.

Perforations, ulcerations and bleedings

Gastric perforation, ulceration and bleeding (PUB) are the most serious and life-threatening side effects associated with NSAID treatment. Although relatively rare, the widespread use of NSAIDs makes them a significant clinical and economic problem. The occurrence of PUB side effects over time in double-blind studies of patients with osteoarthritis or rheumatoid arthritis are illustrated in the incidence curves shown in Figure 4. Both doses of meloxicam were associated with a significantly ($p < 0.05$) lower risk of PUBs than piroxicam and naproxen. The incidence of PUBs with diclofenac (recognized as one of the safer NSAIDs with respect to perforation, bleeding and other serious gastrointestinal events) was greater than with either dose of meloxicam, although the difference did not achieve statistical significance.

As expected, PUBs occurred more frequently overall in patients aged over 65 years than in younger patients[11]. However, there were no PUBs in patients over 65 years old treated with meloxicam 7.5 mg. Similarly, the incidence of PUBs in patients over 65 years old who were treated with meloxicam 15 mg was lower than in patients treated

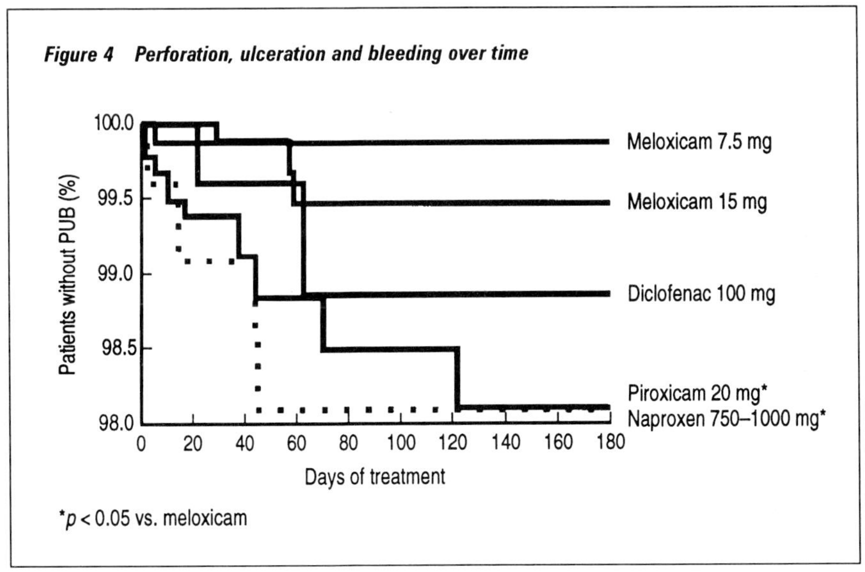

with piroxicam, diclofenac or naproxen. Naproxen was associated with a considerably higher risk than any of the other NSAIDs.

Renal function

Significantly abnormal renal function was defined as serum creatinine > 1.8 mg/dl or blood urea nitrogen values > 40 mg/dl associated with serum creatinine values above the upper limit of normal, with values recorded during treatment higher than those at baseline.

In the global safety analysis of all patients, significantly abnormal renal function was experienced by only 0.4% of patients treated with 7.5 mg or 15 mg meloxicam. This was comparable to the incidence seen with diclofenac SR (0.3%) and naproxen (0.4%). However, the incidence was somewhat higher with piroxicam (0.9%).

CONCLUSIONS

The efficacy of meloxicam (7.5 mg and 15 mg) has been compared with the established NSAIDs, piroxicam (20 mg), diclofenac (100 mg SR) and naproxen (750 mg) in eight large double-blind studies conducted in over 3700 patients with osteoarthritis or rheumatoid arthritis. Both short-term and long term studies were included in this clinical data package and the efficacy of meloxicam was shown to be comparable to that of the other established NSAIDs in all eight studies.

The global safety analysis of meloxicam in comparison with other NSAIDs has involved a total of 5648 patients, 3727 of whom were osteoarthritis or rheumatoid arthritis patients enrolled in double-blind studies. Findings from this analysis confirmed the good safety and tolerability profile of meloxicam. Both doses of meloxicam (7.5 mg and 15 mg) were associated with a lower overall incidence of adverse events than diclofenac SR and naproxen and a similar incidence to piroxicam. As gastrointestinal side effects are the major problem associated with NSAIDs, it is important to note that the gastrointestinal safety profile of meloxicam (7.5 mg and 15 mg) was markedly better than that of any of the other comparator NSAIDs (naproxen, diclofenac SR or piroxicam). This may be due to the preferential inhibition of COX-2 over COX-1 by meloxicam. Meloxicam was associated with a low incidence of renal side effects, comparable with diclofenac SR and naproxen. In contrast, piroxicam was associated with a considerably higher incidence than any of the other NSAIDs.

In conclusion, meloxicam has proven comparable efficacy to the other established therapies for the treatment of osteoarthritis and rheumatoid arthritis and, in addition, has superior tolerability with respect to gastrointestinal side effects.

References

1. Türck D, Busch U, Heinzel G, Narjes H. Clinical pharmacokinetics of meloxicam. Eur J Rheumatol Inflam. 1996;15:in press.
2. Patoia L, Santucci L, Furno P, et al. A 4-week, double-blind, parallel-group study to compare the gastrointestinal effects of meloxicam 7.5 mg, meloxicam 15 mg, piroxicam 20 mg and placebo by means of faecal blood loss, endoscopy and symptoms evaluation in healthy volunteers. Br J Rheumatol. 1996;35(Suppl. 1):61–7.
3. Lund B, Distel M, Bluhmki E. A double-blind, randomized, placebo-controlled study of efficacy and tolerance of meloxicam treatment in patients with osteoarthritis of the knee. Scand J Rheumatol. Submitted.
4. Lindén B, Distel M, Bluhmki E. A double-blind study to compare the efficacy and safety of meloxicam 15 mg with piroxicam 20 mg in patients with osteoarthritis of the hip. Br J Rheumatol. 1996;35(Suppl. 1):35–8.
5. Hosie J, Distel M, Bluhmki E. A six months double-blind study to compare the efficacy, safety and tolerability of meloxicam and piroxicam in patients with osteoarthritis of the hip or knee. Clin Drug Invest. Submitted.
6. Goei Thé H, Lund B, Distel M, Bluhmki E. A double-blind, randomised trial to compare meloxicam 15 mg with diclofenac 100 mg in the treatment of osteoarthritis of the knee. Osteoarthritis Cartilage. Submitted.
7. Hosie J, Distel M, Bluhmki E. Meloxicam in osteoarthritis: a 6-month, double-blind comparison with diclofenac sodium. Br J Rheumatol. 1996;35(Suppl. 1):39–43.
8. Lemmel EM, Bolten W, Bourgos-Vargas R, et al. A double-blind, randomized placebo controlled trial to evaluate the efficacy and safety of meloxicam 7.5 mg and 15 mg once-daily in patients with rheumatoid arthritis. J Rheumatol. Submitted.
9. Huskisson EC, Narjes H, Bluhmki E. A 3-week double-blind, randomised multicentre trial comparing the efficacy and tolerability of meloxicam, a new NSAID, in daily doses of 15 and 30 mg with piroxicam 20 mg in rheumatoid arthritis. Eur J Rheumatol Inflamm. Submitted.
10. Wojtulewski JA, Schattenkirchner M, Barceló P, et al. A six months double-blind trial to compare the efficacy and safety of meloxicam 7.5 mg daily and naproxen 750 mg daily in patients with rheumatoid arthritis. Br J Rheumatol. 1996;35(Suppl. 1):22–8.
11. Distel M, Mueller C, Bluhmki E, Fries J. Safety of meloxicam: a global analysis of clinical trials. Br J Rheumatol. 1996;35(Suppl. 1):68–77.

13 Enzymatic regulation of the prostaglandin response in a human model of inflammation

B. F. McADAM and G. A. FITZGERALD

Prostaglandins (PG) are potent biological mediators of thrombosis and the inflammatory response[1,2]. Prostaglandin endoperoxide H synthase, also referred to as cyclooxygenase (COX), is a bisfunctional protein, which catalyses the first committed step in the formation of PG and thromboxanes by the sequential cyclooxygenation and peroxidation of arachidonic acid (AA) to PGH_2[3,4]. PGH_2 is then converted to specific PGs by distinct cell specific synthases or isomerases. Mammalian cells contain two isoforms of this enzyme, COX-1 and COX-2, which are encoded by separate genes, but they are structurally homologous and have similar kinetic properties[5-7].

COX-1 is expressed constitutively in almost all tissues. Products of this pathway are thought to mediate physiological effects such as vascular homeostasis and gastroprotection in response to circulating hormones. COX-2 is undetectable in the absence of activation in most cells, except in some specialized tissues such as brain, testis and macula densa[8,9]. It is, however, an immediate early gene which is readily induced in response to cytokines, growth factors, phorbol esters and bacterial lipopolysaccharide (LPS)[10-12]. This isoform is expressed in monocytes, macrophages and endothelial cells at sites of inflammation. COX-2 expression is inhibited by glucocorticoids both in vitro and in vivo and by anti-inflammatory cytokines, such as IL-4 and IL-10[13,14].

These observations formed the basis for the assumption that COX-2 expression mediates the enhanced prostanoid release which characterizes the inflammatory response. Such a rationale underlines the development of selective COX-inhibitors. This hypothesis was reinforced by several investigators who demonstrated that increased PG formation, coincident with the induction of COX-2, was blocked by selective COX-2 inhibitors in in vitro systems and in animal models of inflammation in vivo[15,16]. Studies of COX gene inactivation in mice suggest that the role of these isoforms in integrated biological systems may be more complex than hitherto appreciated[17,18]. To examine the biological roles of these enzymes in human disease we have developed a human model of acute inflammation, using the controlled administration of bacterial LPS to healthy volunteers[19-21].

Endotoxin, the LPS outer membrane constituent of Gram-negative bacteria, is well recognized for its ability to activate the immune system and to elicit a wide range of responses in vivo. These are mediated by the elaboration of a cascade of pro-inflammatory effector molecules, including prostanoids and cytokines, and activation of the fibrinolytic and coagulation pathways[22-24]. The functional importance of the prostanoid response is emphasized by the finding that prior administration of aspirin and other non steroid anti-inflammatory drugs (NSAIDs) significantly attenuates many of the systemic responses induced by LPS[25,26].

STUDY DESIGN

Nine male and nine female volunteers passed a screen for study eligibility at the Clinical Research Center (CRC) in the Hospital of the University of Pennsylvania. The study was scrutinized and approved by the Institutional Review Board. Volunteers were randomized, under double blind conditions, to receive a bolus injection of a saline control or endotoxin at a dose of either 2 ng/kg or 4 ng/kg. The endotoxin preparation used was Food and Drug Administration US Reference *Escherichia coli* endotoxin lot EC-5, kindly provided by Dr H.D. Hochstein, Bureau of Biologics, FDA, Bethesda, MD. This was reconstituted according to FDA prescription.

Urinary eicosanoid metabolites were measured by gas chromatography/mass spectrometry as previously described[27,28].

RESULTS

Clinical

Experimental endotoxaemia produced a characteristic dose–response relationship in terms of the constitutional responses and pyrexia. The protocol was well tolerated by the volunteers. A 'flu-like syndrome was induced within 2–3 h, consisting of fever, headache, malaise, myalgia and fatigue. Figure 1 shows the time course of the temperature response to LPS, which peaked at 4 h. A hyperdynamic cardiovascular response was observed with significant increases in heart rate, but with minor changes in blood pressure. A characteristic stress hormone response was observed with an early rise in plasma cortisol compared with the normal diurnal variation observed in volunteers who received placebo (Figure 2). Most parameters returned to normal by 8–10 h after LPS administration.

Urinary metabolites

The kinetics of systemic biosynthesis of eicosanoids in response to LPS were examined. There was a dramatic increase in the excretion of a major metabolite of thromboxane (Tx-M), 11-dehydrothromboxane B_2, coincident with the onset of constitutional symptoms in volunteers who experienced a pyrexial response. This peaked in the first 6 h. There was no change in the capacity of blood to produce thromboxane, as levels of serum thromboxane B_2 remained unchanged. LPS also caused a dose-dependent increase in prostacyclin biosynthesis, the major eicosanoid produced by endothelial cells, as reflected in the elevated levels of its major metabolite in urine, 2,3-dinor-6-keto $PGF_{1\alpha}$ (PGI-M) (Figure 3).

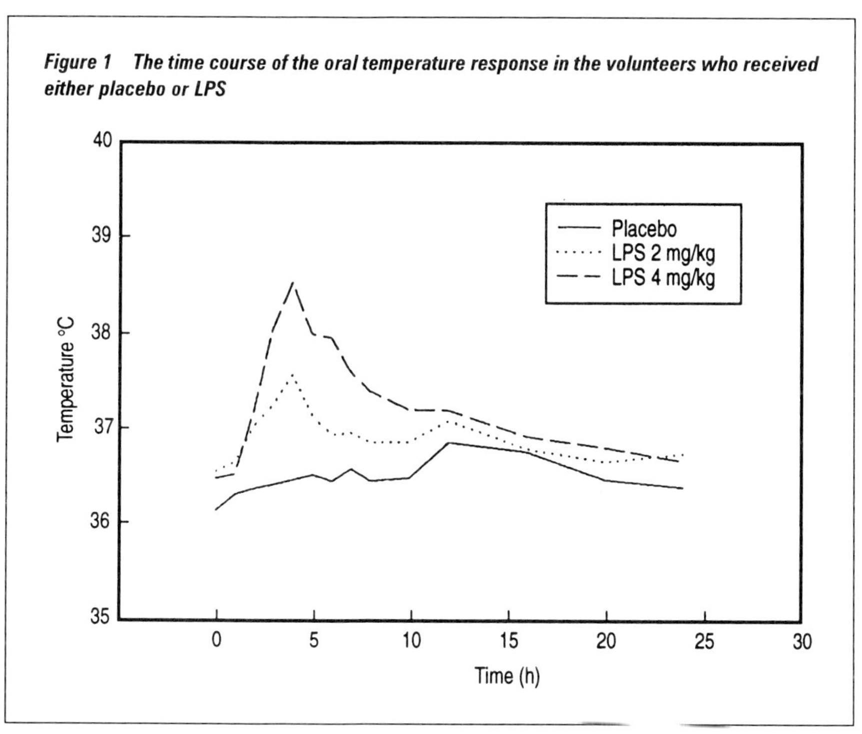

Figure 1 **The time course of the oral temperature response in the volunteers who received either placebo or LPS**

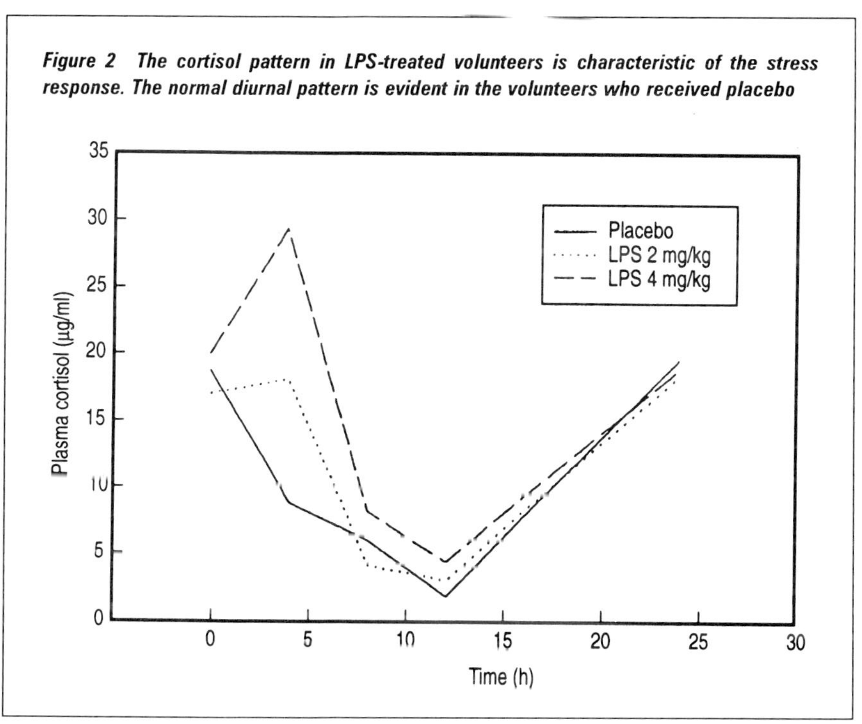

Figure 2 **The cortisol pattern in LPS-treated volunteers is characteristic of the stress response. The normal diurnal pattern is evident in the volunteers who received placebo**

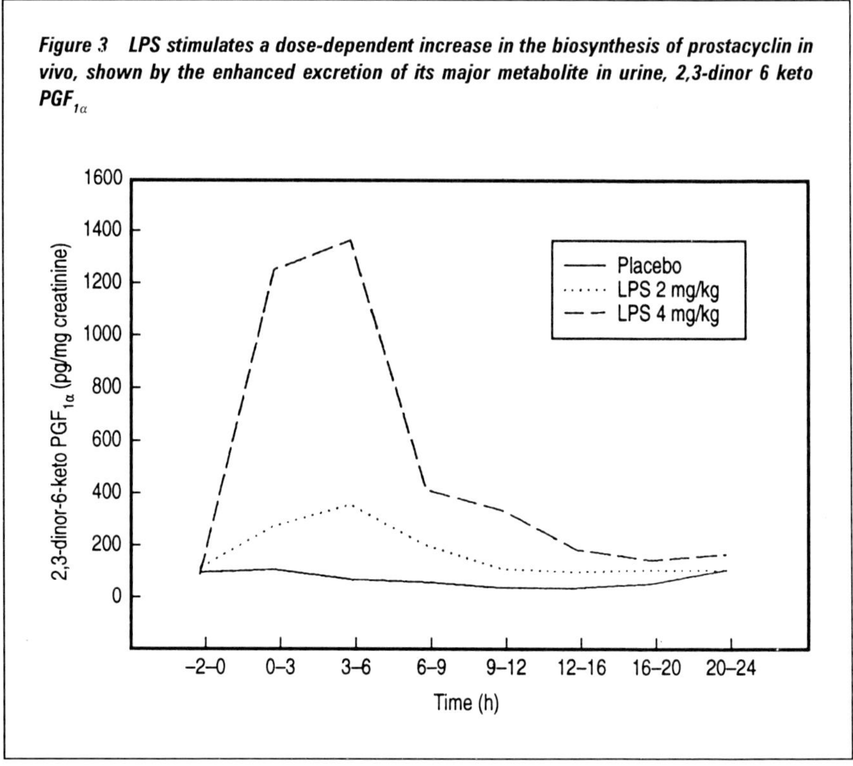

Figure 3 *LPS stimulates a dose-dependent increase in the biosynthesis of prostacyclin in vivo, shown by the enhanced excretion of its major metabolite in urine, 2,3-dinor 6 keto PGF$_{1\alpha}$*

DISCUSSION

The decision to develop sensitive COX-2 inhibitors is based on the assumption that COX-2 induction is responsible for prostaglandin generation in inflammatory states, whereas COX-1 activity serves a more physiological function. The side effects of currently available NSAIDs, which are non-specific with respect to COX inhibition, are considered to be related to inhibition of the constitutively expressed isoform. Thus, it would be anticipated that these toxic effects might be less frequent with selective COX-2 inhibitors. These assumptions have been fundamentally challenged by the results obtained in mice deficient in the COX enzymes: COX-1-deficient mice did not develop GI ulceration, despite an inability to elaborate prostaglandins by gastrointestinal epithelial cells. They did, however, exhibit an impaired early inflammatory response which was not seen in COX-2-deficient mice. COX-2-deficient mice, by contrast, were capable of mounting an inflammatory response (peritonitis) to incidental infection[17,18].

These observations have provoked a cautious reappraisal of the current hypothesis, not only with respect to the functional role of these isoforms in normal and inflammatory states but also with regard to the mechanistic basis for NSAID gastropathy and renal toxicity. Both isoforms have been isolated in renal tissue, notably in reno-prival states[29].

Further clinical investigation is required to clarify the molecular mechanisms which underlie prostanoid generation during the inflammatory response in vivo. To that end, we have defined a human model of inflammation. Endotoxin has been used to stimulate prostaglandin production in vivo coincident with induction of COX-2 in cell systems and in animal models of inflammation[30,31]. Experimental endotoxaemia in man produces an acute inflammatory response in a dose-dependent but tolerated manner. Using validated indices of eicosanoid biosynthesis, we have characterized the quantitative and qualitative alterations in prostanoid formation in this model of acute inflammation in humans.

To our knowledge, there is only one previous report of the effect of LPS on PG formation in humans. Van der Poll *et al.*[32] demonstrated that LPS (*E. coli* toxin) administered intravenously to three volunteers resulted in an increase of 60% in plasma immunoreactive 6-keto $PGF_{1\alpha}$, the hydrolysis product of prostacyclin (PGI_2), 90 min after injection of 2 ng/kg LPS; levels returned to baseline within 3 h of administration. However, measurements were limited to the first 6 h after endotoxin administration and no other prostanoids were assayed. Moreover potential artifacts involved with this assay method, particularly in a setting where many potential cross-reacting substances were evoked by LPS, make these data difficult to interpret with confidence[33].

In the present study, we observed significant alterations in the biosynthesis of the major metabolites of thromboxane and prostacyclin in vivo, in response to LPS. These increases occurred soon after LPS injection, coinciding with the constitutional and pyrexial response to the lipopolysaccharide.

The kinetics of induction of COX-2 protein (from in vitro studies and animal models of inflammation) do not correlate with either the clinical or predominant eicosanoid biosynthetic response to LPS documented in this study. Interestingly, no late peak in prostaglandin formation, suggestive of delayed induction of COX-2, was apparent after LPS administration.

Many of the biological effects of LPS are mediated through its interaction with peripheral blood monocytes. LPS first complexes with the acute phase protein, LPS binding protein, then binds to CD14 receptors on monocytes, which orchestrate the release of a host of mediator cytokines[34,35]. Monocytes may elaborate prostaglandins either via high levels of expression of the constitutive COX-1 or via their capacity to induce COX-2[36,37].

Given their pivotal role in the inflammatory response, we examined the effect of low dose endotoxin on peripheral blood monocytes isolated from whole blood to help identify the molecular mechanisms which underlie this biosynthetic response in vivo. Expression of COX-1 protein and mRNA, but not COX-2, was readily detectable *ex vivo* in monocytes harvested from volunteers given LPS. These observations imply a contribution of COX-1 to prostaglandin formation in the human inflammatory response. Although they do not rule out a contribution from COX-2, which may have been induced in tissues other than the monocyte, they are consistent with the published experience with COX gene inactivation in vivo.

CONCLUSION

We have demonstrated the feasibility of creating an experimental model of inflammation to characterize the eicosanoid response in humans. This model will improve our understanding of the functional contribution of the two COX isoforms to human inflammation and elucidate the clinical pharmacology of selective COX-2 inhibitors in humans.

Acknowledgements

Supported by a grant from the National Institute of Health (HL 54500).

References

1. FitzGerald GA. Prostaglandins and related compounds. In: Wyngaarden JB, Smith LH, Bennett JC, eds. Cecil Loeb Textbook of Medicine, 20th edn. Philadelphia: Saunders, 1995:1187–93.
2. Smith WL. The eicosanoids and their biochemical mechanisms of action. Biochem J. 1989;259: 315–24.
3. Smith WL, Marnett LJ. Prostaglandin endoperoxide synthase: Structure and catalysis. Biochem Biophys Acta. 1990;1083:1–17.
4. Smith WL. Prostanoid biosynthesis and mechanisms of action. Am J Physiol. 1992;263: F181–91.
5. Hla T, Neilson K. Human cyclooxygenase 2 cDNA. Proc Natl Acad Sci USA. 1992;89:7384–8.
6. O'Bannion MK, Winn VD, Young DA. cDNA Cloning and functional activity of a glucocorticoid-regulated inflammatory cyclooxygenase. Proc Natl Acad Sci USA. 1992;89:4888–92.
7. Hsi LC, Hoganson CW, Babcock GT, Smith WL. Characterization of a tyrosyl radical in prostaglandin endoperoxide synthase-2. Biochem Biophys Res Commun. 1994;202:1592–8.
8. Yamagata K, Andreasson K, Kaufmann W, Barnes CA, Worley PF. Expression of a mitogen inducible cyclooxygenase in brain neurons: regulation by synaptic activity and glucocorticoids. Neuron. 1993;11:371–86.
9. O'Neill GP, Ford-Hutchinson AW. Expression of mRNA for cyclooxygenase-1 and cyclo-oxygenase-2 in human tissues. FEBS Lett. 1993;330:156–60.
10. Fu JY, Masferrer JL, Seibert K, Raz A, Needleman P. The induction and suppression of prosta-glandin H_2 synthase (cyclooxygenase) in human monocytes. J Biol Chem. 1990;265:16737–40.
11. Masferrer JL, Zweifel BS, Seibert K, Needleman P. Selective regulation of cellular cyclooxy-genase by dexamethasone and endotoxin in mice. J Clin Invest. 1990;86:1375–9.
12. Crofford LJ, Wilder RL, Ristimaki AP, Sano H, Remmers EF, Epps HR, Hla T. Cyclooxygenase-1 and -2 expression in rheumatoid synovial tissues. J Clin Invest. 1994;93:1095–101.
13. Masferrer JL, Srinivasa TR, Zweifel BS, Seibert K, Needleman P, Gilbert RS, Herschman HR. *In vivo* glucocorticoids regulate cyclooxygenase-1 but not cyclooxygenase-1 in peritoneal macrophages. J Pharmacol Exp Ther. 1994;270:1340–4.
14. Mertz PM, DeWitt DL, Steller-Stevenson WG, Wahl LM. Interleukin 10 suppression of monocyte prostaglandin H synthase-2. J Biol Chem. 1994;269:21322–9.
15. Seibert K, Zhang Y, Leahy K, Hauser S, Masferrer J, Perkins W, Lee L, Isakson PC. Pharmaco-logical and biochemical demonstration of the role of cyclooxygenase 2 in inflammation and pain. Proc Natl Acad Sci USA. 1994;91:12013–17.
16. Masferrer JL, Zweifel BS, Manning PT, Hauser S, Leahy KM, Smith WG, Isakson PC, Seibert K. Selective inhibition of inducible cyclooxygenase 2 in vivo is antiinflammatory and nonulcerogenic. Proc Natl Acad Sci USA. 1994;91:3228–32.
17. Morham SC, Langenbach R, Loftin CD, Tiano HF *et al.* Prostaglandin synthase 2 gene disruption causes severe renal pathology in the mouse. Cell. 1995;83:473–82.
18. Langenbach R, Morham SG, Tiano HF, Loftin CD, *et al.* Prostaglandin synthase 1 gene disruption in mice reduces arachidonic acid-induced inflammation and indomethacin-induced gastric ulceration. Cell. 1995;83:483–92.

19. Martich GD, Boujoukos AJ, Suffredini AF. Response of man to endotoxin. Immunobiology. 1993;187:403–16.
20. Suffredini AF, Fromm E, Parker MM *et al.* The cardiovascular response of normal humans to the administration of endotoxin. N Engl J Med. 1989;321:280–7.
21. Michie HR, Maogue PC, Spriggs DR, Revhaug A *et al.* Detection of circulating tumour necrosis factor after endotoxin administration. N Engl J Med. 1988;318:1481–6.
22. Cassale TB, Ballas ZK, Kaliner MA, Keahey TM. The effects of intravenous endotoxin on various host effector molecules. J Allergy Clin Immunol. 1990;85:45–51.
23. Suffredini AF, Harpel PC, Parrillo JE. Promotion and subsequent inhibition of plasminogen activator after administration of intravenous endotoxin to normal subjects. N Engl J Med. 1989; 320:1165–72.
24. Rodrick ML, Moss NM, Grbic JT *et al.* Effects of endotoxin infusions on the in vitro cellular immune responses in humans. J Clin Immunol. 1992;12:440–50.
25. Spinas GA, Bloesch D, Keller U, Zimmerli W, Cammisuli S. Pretreatment with ibuprofen augments circulating tumour necrosis factor α, interleukin-6, and elastase during acute endotoxaemia. J Infect Dis. 1991;163:89–95.
26. Martich GD, Parker MM, Cunnion RE, Suffredini AF. Effects of ibuprofen and pentoxifylline on the cardiovascular response of normal humans to endotoxin. J Appl Physiol. 1992;73:925–31.
27. FitzGerald GA, Brash AR, Blair IA, Lawson J. Analysis of urinary metabolites of thromboxane and prostacyclin by negative ion chemical ionization gas chromatography-mass spectrometry. In: Hayaishi O, Yamamoto S, eds. Advances in Prostaglandin, Thromboxane and Leukotriene Research. New York: Raven Press, 1985:87–90.
28. Catella F, Johnson JM, FitzGerald GA. Quantitative analysis of eicosanoids by gas chromatography-mass spectrometry. In: Samuelsson BB, Berti F, Folco G, Velo GP, editors. Prostanoids and Drugs. New York: Plenum Press (NATO ASI Series). 1989:15–22.
29. Harris RC, McKanna JA, Akai Y, Jacobson HR, Dubois RN, Breyer MD. Cyclooxygenase 2 is associated with the macula densa of rat kidney and increases with salt restriction. J Clin Invest. 1994;94.2504–10.
30. O'Sullivan MG, Huggins EM, Meade EA, DeWitt D, McCall CE. Lipopolysaccharide induces prostaglandin H synthase 2 in alveolar macrophages. Biochem Biophys Res Commun. 1992; 187:1123–7.
31. Lee SH, Soyoola E, Chanmugam P, Hart S, *et al.* Selective expression of mitogen inducible cyclooxygenase in macrophages stimulated with lipopolysaccharide. J Biol Chem. 1992;267: 25934–8.
32. Van der Poll T, Van Deventer SJ, Buller HR, *et al.* Comparison of the early dynamics of systemic prostacyclin release after administration of tumour necrosis factor and endotoxin to healthy humans. J Infect Dis. 1991;164:599–601.
33. Pedersen AK, Watson M, FitzGerald GA. Inhibition of thromboxane synthase in serum: limitations of the measurement of immunoreactive 6 keto-PGF$_{1\alpha}$. Thrombosis Res. 1983;33:99–103.
34. Wright SD, Ramos PS, Tobias RJ, Ulevitch RJ, Mathison JC. CD14, a receptor for complexes of lipopolysaccharide (LPS) and LPS binding protein. Science. 190;249:1431.
35. Leeuwenberg JF, Dentener MA, Buurman WA. Lipopolysaccharide LPS-mediated soluble TNR receptor release and TNF receptor expression by monocytes. J Immunol. 1994;152:5070–6.
36. Vane JR, Botting RM. A better understanding of anti-inflammatory drugs based on isoforms of cyclooxygenase (COX-1 and COX-2). Adv Pros Thromb Leuk Res. 1995;23:41–8.
37. Hempel SL, Monick MM, Hunninghake GW. Lipopolysaccharide induces prostaglandin H synthase 2 protein and mRNA in human alveolar macrophages and blood monocytes. J Clin Invest. 1994;93:391–6.

14 Cyclooxygenase-2 and intestinal cancer

R. N. DUBOIS, A. RADHIKA, J. SHAO, M. TSUJII,
H. SHENG, O. KOBYASHI, R. D. BEAUCHAMP and
C. S. WILLIAMS

Multiple epidemiological studies reveal a 40–50% reduction in mortality from colorectal cancer in individuals taking non-steroid anti-inflammatory drugs (NSAIDs) on a regular basis compared with those not taking these agents[1-6]. Persons with familial adenomatous polyposis (FAP) who take sulindac show a striking reduction in adenoma size and number[7-11]. In rodent models of azoxymethane-induced colorectal carcinogenesis, cyclooxygenase (COX) inhibitors exhibit chemoprotective effects as judged by a reduction in the frequency and number of premalignant and malignant lesions[12-14]. Recently, Jacoby et al.[15] reported a decrease in tumour number in Min (multiple intestinal neoplasia) mice treated with piroxicam.

The mechanism by which NSAIDs reduce the risk of colorectal neoplasia or cause tumour regression is unknown. One possibility involves altered metabolism of arachidonic acid, since NSAIDs inhibit COX enzymes, thereby reducing eicosanoid production. Products of the COX pathway appear to modulate numerous signal transduction pathways in a variety of cell types[16]. Some investigators have noted elevated levels of prostaglandins (PG) in colorectal carcinomas compared to normal mucosa[17,18]. Therefore, it seems plausible that the COX pathway of arachidonic acid metabolism may be involved in this chemoprotective effect of NSAIDs. Other effects of NSAIDs (non-COX mediated) have been reported and at higher concentrations, these compounds can induce programmed cell death directly in cultured cells[19,20]. The effects seen at high doses are not likely to be related to the ability of these compounds to inhibit COX, since compounds which cause little or no inhibition (sulindac sulfone) induce apoptosis in HT-29 cells when given at concentrations ranging from 0.50 to 0.75 mM[21]. Since HT-29 cells are said to express very low or even undetectable levels of the COX enzymes, the chemoprotective effects of therapeutic doses of NSAIDs are probably due to their action on the COX pathway.

At least two cyclooxygenase isoforms have been identified, cyclooxygenase-1 (COX-1) and cyclooxygenase-2 (COX-2). COX-1 is constitutively expressed under most circumstances, whereas COX-2 is induced by cytokines, growth factors and tumour promoters[22]. Our laboratory has shown that COX-2 expression is induced in non-transformed intestinal epithelial cells by transforming growth factor-α (TGFα)[23]. We have also recently demonstrated that intestinal epithelial cells overexpressing the COX-2 gene develop altered adhesion properties and are resistant to the process of programmed cell death[24]. Both of these phenotypic changes are reversed by treatment

Table 1   Phenotypic changes associated with COX-2 expression in RIE-1 cells

Phenotypic change	RIE-P	RIE-AS	RIE-S
Length of G_1 cell cycle phase (h)	10–12	8–10	20–24
Adhesion to laminin	+/–	+/–	++++
Na butyrate-induced apoptosis	+++	++++	+/–

RIE-P, parental RIE cells; RIE-AS, RIE cells permanently transfected with the antisense COX-2 expression vector; RIE-S, RIE cells permanently transfected with the sense COX-2 expression vector

Table 2   Biochemical changes associated with COX-2 expression in RIE-1 cells

Biochemical parameter	RIE-P	RIE-AS	RIE-S
Cyclin D1 levels	+++	+++	+/–
Bcl-2 levels	–	–	++++
E-cadherin	+++	+++	–
TGFβ type II Receptor	+++	+++	+/–

RIE-P, parental RIE cells; RIE-AS, RIE cells permanently transfected with the antisense COX-2 expression vector; RIE-S, RIE cells permanently transfected with the sense COX-2 expression vector

with low levels of NSAIDs (1–50 μM). Overexpression of COX-2 may therefore alter the tumorigenic potential of intestinal epithelial cells. The sensitivity of the two COX isoforms to NSAID inhibition differs[25,26] and this enables targeting of COX-2 in chemoprevention strategies, if this isoform is proven to be involved in colorectal carcinogenesis.

COX-2 IN INTESTINAL EPITHELIAL CELLS

To investigate the possible role of COX-2 overexpression in colorectal cancer, we prepared an in vitro model in which parental rat intestinal epithelial cells (RIE-P) were permanently transfected with a COX-2 expression vector oriented in the sense (RIE-S) or antisense (RIE-AS) direction. COX-2 protein and enzyme activity were at least 10 to 20-fold higher in the RIE-S cells than in the RIE-AS cells. We observed a number of phenotypic changes in RIE-S cells, which overexpress COX-2 (see Table 1). In particular, they attach to components of the extracellular matrix (ECM) (e.g. laminin) with greater avidity than cells which do not express this enzyme, they resist undergoing apoptosis when stimulated to do so and they have a prolonged G_1 phase of the cell cycle. We also demonstrated biochemical changes in RIE cells overexpressing the COX-2 gene (see Table 2). The RIE-S cells express higher levels of Bcl-2 and lower levels of cyclin D1, transforming growth factor-β (TGFβ) type II receptor and E-cadherin. These changes could enhance the tumorigenic potential of intestinal epithelial cells. Since COX-2 expression levels increase dramatically in colorectal cancer (see Table 3), our findings may relate to the ability of cyclooxygenase inhibitors, such as aspirin and other NSAIDs, to reduce the relative risk of colorectal cancer in humans.

The results of our work suggests that COX-2 overexpression may alter intestinal

Table 3   NSAIDs. COX and colorectal cancer

| | | | COX-2 level | |
| | | | Tumour | Normal tissue |
Model	Type	NSAID effect	Tumour	Normal tissue
Human	FAP	Tumour regression	+++	–
Rat	AOM	Decrease in tumour number	++++	–
Min mouse	APC⁻	Decrease in tumour number	+++	–

epithelial biology in a number of ways. Several studies suggest that cell–substrate adhesion may play an important role in tumorigenesis, since cells which have been transformed by a virus or with chemical carcinogens demonstrate altered adhesion to ECM when compared with non-transformed cells. Programmed cell death is one of the most important components in maintaining the integrity of intestinal epithelium. Cellular differentiation and proliferative arrest are induced as intestinal stem cells ascend upward on basement membrane along the crypt–villus axis toward the intestinal lumen. When the cells reach the surface of the villi they become fully differentiated, undergo programmed cell death and are shed into the lumen. The life of an epithelial cell in humans is only 4–5 days. Factors which could prolong cell survival could influence the integrity and function of intestinal mucosa. Prolonged cell survival and increased adhesion to matrix components could also have significant biological consequences and affect the tumorigenic potential of epithelial cells. The study of apoptosis has become the focus of a number of groups evaluating the molecular basis for the development of colorectal cancer. Prolonged survival of abnormal cells can favour tumour progression and facilitate the accumulation of sequential genetic mutations which would result in tumour promotion. In the context of intestinal epithelium in vivo, high COX-2 levels would increase the time that abnormal cells (with a primary mutation) would spend in transit to the villus tip and increase the chance that a second mutation could occur (tumour progression). Our results are consistent with this hypothesis, demonstrating that RIE-S cells have prolonged survival under conditions in which apoptosis is normally induced. They also support a protective role of NSAIDs, since following inhibition of cyclooxygenase the cells undergo programmed cell death quite readily.

The effect of COX-2 overexpression on TGFβ type II receptor and E-cadherin expression levels could also play a significant role in tumorigenesis (see Table 2). TGFβ inhibits the growth of epithelial cells, and some reports have indicated that loss of this negative regulation contributes to colorectal tumour development. The TGFβ growth inhibitory signal is transduced through two receptors. TGFβ type I (RI) and TGFβ type II (RII). TGFβ RII transcripts were undetectable or present at markedly reduced amounts in some human colon cancer cell lines, although TGFβ RI transcripts were detected in all samples. Reduced TGFβ RII receptor expression, by inducing the escape of cells from TGFβ-mediated growth control, would also increase the probability that cells expressing high COX-2 levels would have prolonged survival and therefore be at risk for tumour progression. Local invasion is thought to be one of the most important factors for tumour formation. Some reports have shown that more than

80% of poorly differentiated tumours lack expression of E-cadherin. These results suggest that the presence of E-cadherin is important in cell differentiation and that down-regulation of E-cadherin expression is associated with local invasion of tumour cells.

DISCUSSION

Understanding of the molecular events involved in the development of colorectal neoplasia has progressed remarkably during the past decade. Recent clinical and epidemiological studies have shown an inverse relationship between NSAID use and colorectal cancer risk in humans[1-6]. Although the mechanisms whereby NSAIDs mediate these effects are unknown, inhibition of COX, leading to a reduction of eicosanoid production, remains a possibility. We and others have shown that mitogen-inducible COX-2 expression is up-regulated in human colorectal carcinomas[27-29].

Colorectal cancer is the second leading cause of death from cancer in the United States. In early stages of the disease a cure is possible, but unfortunately these malignancies have often grown beyond the large intestine by the time they are detected and our current treatment regimens are not very effective. Work carried out by several basic science groups over the last decade has focused on the molecular basis of colorectal cancer and tremendous progress has been made. Clinical investigators have observed a 40–50% reduction in the relative risk of colorectal cancer in humans who take NSAIDs (like aspirin) on a regular basis. One of the molecular targets for NSAIDs is COX. Our work presented here demonstrates that when intestinal epithelial cells overexpress COX-2 they adhere more avidly to extracellular matrix proteins and they are resistant to apoptosis. Both of these phenotypic changes are reversed by the addition of a COX inhibitor (sulindac). These results may provide some insight regarding the molecular basis for the chemoprotective effects of NSAIDs. The relationship between regional location of the lesion in the colon and COX-2 expression may also be extremely important, since one recent report indicates that chemopreventive agents may be more protective against right-sided lesions[30] than against left-sided colonic tumours. Studies are also underway to determine whether tumours which develop in animals being treated with NSAIDs lack expression of this enzyme.

Acknowledgements

This work was supported in part by funds from the A.B. Hancock, Jr. Memorial Laboratory (R.N.D.), Lucille P. Markey Charitable Trust (R.N.D.) and the United States Public Health Services Grants NIHES 00267 (R.N.D.), DK 47297-02 (R.N.D.). R.N.D. is the recipient of a VA Research Associate career development award, Boehringer Ingelheim New Investigator Award, and is an AGA Industry Research Scholar.

References

1. Giovannucci E, Egan KM, Hunter DJ et al. Aspirin and the risk of colorectal cancer in women. N Engl J Med. 1995;333:609–14.
2. Greenberg ER, Baron JA, Freeman DHJ, Mandel JS, Haile R. Reduced risk of large-bowel

adenomas among aspirin users. The Polyp Prevention Study Group. J Natl Cancer Inst. 1993;85: 912–16.

3. Thun MJ, Namboodiri MM, Heath CWJ. Aspirin use and reduced risk of fatal colon cancer. N Engl J Med. 1991;325:1593–6.

4. Thun MJ, Namboodiri MM, Calle EE, Flanders WD, Heath CWJ. Aspirin use and risk of fatal cancer. Cancer Res. 1993;53:1322–7.

5. Peleg II, Maibach HT, Brown SH, Wilcox CM. Aspirin and nonsteroidal anti-inflammatory drug use and the risk of subsequent colorectal cancer. Arch Intern Med. 1994;154:394–9.

6. Giovannucci E, Rimm EB, Stampfer MJ, Colditz GA, Ascherio A, Willett WC. Aspirin use and the risk for colorectal cancer and adenoma in male health professionals. Ann Intern Med. 1994; 121:241–6.

7. Giardiello FM, Hamilton SR, Krush AJ et al. Treatment of colonic and rectal adenomas with sulindac in familial adenomatous polyposis. N Engl J Med. 1993;328:1313–16.

8. Waddell WR, Loughry RW. Sulindac for polyposis of the colon. J Surg Oncol. 1983;24:83–7.

9. Waddell WR, Gasner GF, Cerise EJ, Loughry RW. Sulindac for polyposis of the colon. Am J Surg. 1989;157:175–8.

10. Winde G, Gumbinger HG, Osswald H, Kemper F, Bunte H. The NSAID sulindac reverses rectal adenomas in colectomized patients with familial adenomatous polyposis: clinical results of a dose-finding study on rectal sulindac administration. Int J Colorectal Dis. 1993;8:13–17.

11. Nugent KP, Farmer KC, Spigelman AD, Williams CB, Phillips RK. Randomized controlled trial of the effect of sulindac on duodenal and rectal polyposis and cell proliferation in patients with familial adenomatous polyposis. Br J Surg. 1993;80:1618–19.

12. Reddy BS, Nayini J, Tokumo K, Rigotty J, Zang E, Kelloff G. Chemoprevention of colon carcinogenesis by concurrent administration of piroxicam, a nonsteroidal antiinflammatory drug with D,L-alpha-difluoromethylornithine, an ornithine decarboxylase inhibitor, in diet. Cancer Res. 1990;50:2562–8.

13. Reddy BS, Rao CV, Rivenson A, Kelloff G. Inhibitor effect of aspirin on azoxymethane-induced colon carcinogenesis in F344 rats. Carcinogenesis. 1993;14:1493–7.

14. Craven PA, DeRubertis FR. Effects of aspirin on 1,2-dimethylhydrazine-induced colonic carcinogenesis. Carcinogenesis. 1992;13:541–6.

15. Jacoby RF, Marshall DJ, Newton MA et al. Chemoprevention of spontaneous intestinal adenomas in the Apc^{Min} mouse model by the nonsteroidal anti-inflammatory drug piroxicam. Cancer Res. 1996;56:710–14.

16. Eberhart CE, DuBois RN. Eicosanoids and the gastrointestinal tract. Gastroenterology. 1995;109: 285–301.

17. Rigas B, Goldman IS, Levine L. Altered eicosanoid levels in human colon cancer. J Lab Clin Med. 1993;122:518–23.

18. Rao CV, Rivenson A, Simi B et al. Chemoprevention of colon carcinogenesis by sulindac, a nonsteroidal anti-inflammatory agent. Cancer Res. 1995;55:1464–72.

19. Shiff SJ, Qiao L, Tsai LL, Rigas B. Sulindac sulfide, an aspirin-like compound, inhibits proliferation, causes cell cycle quiescence, and induces apoptosis in HT-29 colon adenocarcinoma cells. J Clin Invest. 1995;96:491–503.

20. Lu X, Xie W, Reed D, Bradshaw WS, Simmons DL. Nonsteroidal antiinflammatory drugs cause apoptosis and induce cyclooxygenase in chicken embryo fibroblasts. Proc Natl Acad Sci USA. 1995;92:7961–5.

21. Piazza GA, Rahm AL, Krutzsch M et al. Antineoplastic drugs sulindac sulfide and sulfone inhibit cell growth by inducing apoptosis. Cancer Res. 1995;55:3110–16.

22. Williams CW, DuBois RN. Prostaglandin endoperoxide synthase: why two isoforms? Am J Physiol. 1996;270:G393–G400.

23. DuBois RN, Awad J, Morrow J, Roberts LJ, Bishop PR. Regulation of eicosanoid production and mitogenesis in rat intestinal epithelial cells by transforming growth factor-α and phorbol ester. J Clin Invest. 1994;93:493–8.

24. Tsujii M, DuBois RN. Alterations in cellular adhesion and apoptosis in epithelial cells overexpressing prostaglandin endoperoxide synthase-2. Cell. 1995;83:493–501.

25. Meade EA, Smith WL, DeWitt DL. Differential inhibition of prostaglandin endoperoxide synthase (cyclooxygenase) isozymes by aspirin and other non-steroidal anti-inflammatory drugs. J Biol Chem. 1993;268:6610–14.

26. Masferrer JL, Zweifel BS, Manning PT et al. Selective inhibition of inducible cyclooxygenase-2 in vivo is antiinflammatory and nonulcerogenic. Proc Natl Acad Sci USA. 1994;91:3228–32.
27. Eberhart CE, Coffey RJ, Radhika A, Giardiello FM, Ferrenbach S, DuBois RN. Up-regulation of cyclooxygenase 2 gene expression in human colorectal adenomas and adenocarcinomas. Gastroenterology. 1994;107:1183–8.
28. Kargman S, O'Neill G, Vickers P, Evans J, Mancini J, Jothy S. Expression of prostaglandin G/H synthase-1 and -2 protein in human colon cancer. Cancer Res. 1995;55:2556–9.
29. Sano H, Kawahito Y, Wilder RL et al. Expression of cyclooxygenase-1 and -2 in human colorectal cancer. Cancer Res. 1995;55:3785–9.
30. Liu T, Mikuolu AO, Rao CV, Reddy BS, Holt PR. Regional chemoprevention of carcinogen-induced tumors in rat colon. Gastroenterology. 1995;109:1167–72.

15 Cytokines and adhesion molecules in the lung inflammatory response

P. A. WARD

Intrapulmonary deposition of IgG immune complexes in rat lung triggers a series of inflammatory responses that result in acute lung injury involving vascular endothelial cells, alveolar epithelial cells and connective tissue matrix. Understanding of these pathophysiological events may yield information for human inflammatory diseases such as rheumatoid arthritis, systemic lupus erythematosus, membranous nephritis and systemic vasculitis, all of which are characterized by deposition of IgG immune complexes together with complement activation products. The IgG immune complex model of acute lung injury in rats is triggered by the airway instillation of rabbit polyclonal antibody (IgG) against bovine serum albumin (BSA) followed by the intravenous infusion of BSA. The inflammatory response (neutrophil accumulation) and evidence of injury (leakage of [125I]albumin and haemorrhage) reaches a maximum at 4h and then, for reasons not fully understood, undergoes remission. The availability of complement and the accumulation of neutrophils are central to the development of injury. Adhesion molecules, both on endothelial cells and on leukocytes themselves, play an important role in the inflammatory outcome.

ROLE OF OXIDANTS

Injury to the lung parenchyma in this model can be most directly linked to the role of NADPH oxidase of neutrophils and macrophages as well as participation of inducible nitric oxide synthase (iNOS) (Figure 1). The former enzyme is activated by assembly of an oxidase complex on the surface of phagocytic cells, resulting in generation of superoxide anion (O_2^-), H_2O_2 and the hydroxyl radical ($HO^\cdot$). In this inflammatory model expression of iNOS in lung involves both alveolar macrophages and alveolar Type II epithelial cells. In vivo expression of iNOS requires three cytokines: tumour necrosis factor-α (TNFα), interleukin 1 (IL-1) and interferon-γ (IFNγ)[1]. Oxidant products of iNOS include nitric oxide ($NO^\cdot$), its reaction product with O_2^-, peroxynitric anion ($ONOO^-$), and $HO^\cdot$ as well as nitrate and nitrite. The most reactive oxidants are $HO^\cdot$ and $ONOO$, which can form adducts on proteins, carbohydrates, lipids and can also cause formation of cross-linked products. Lung injury after deposition of IgG immune complexes is due to a combination of oxidants as well as proteases which are released from neutrophils and macrophages[2]. The relevant proteases are metalloproteinases (e.g. collagenases, gelatinases) and serine proteinases (e.g. elastase,

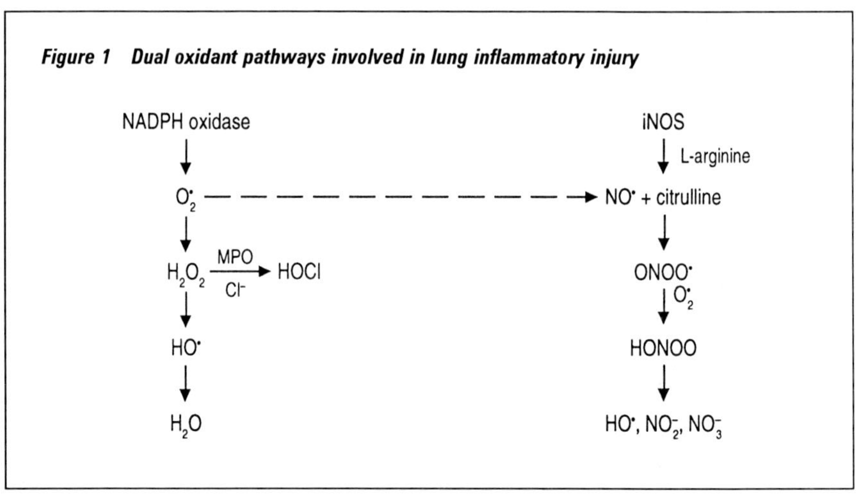

Figure 1   Dual oxidant pathways involved in lung inflammatory injury

cathepsin), as determined by the use of recombinant tissue inhibitor of metallo-proteinase-2 (TIMP-2) and secreted leukocyte protease inhibitor (SLPI)[3].

ROLE OF EARLY RESPONSE CYTOKINES

The key to triggering the lung inflammatory response is production of the 'early response cytokines', $TNF\alpha$ and IL-1 (Figure 2). In the lung, the chief sources of these cytokines are macrophages (alveolar and interstitial), which are activated by contact with immune complexes and complement activation products[4]. Prodigious quantities of these cytokines are released into the bronchoalveolar compartment. Although $TNF\alpha$ and IL-1 have known stimulatory activities for phagocytic cells, it is clear in this inflammatory model that these cytokines are central to the stimulation of endothelial cells, resulting in expression of two important adhesion molecules: E-selectin and intercellular adhesion molecule-1 (ICAM-1). Blockade of either $TNF\alpha$ or IL-1 greatly reduces up-regulation of lung vascular ICAM-1 and E-selectin, substantially reducing recruitment of neutrophils[5]. Similar results have been obtained either by the use of blocking antibodies or by the use of IL-1 receptor antagonist (IL-1Ra) or soluble $TNF\alpha$-R$_I$, the former competing with IL-1 for binding to IL-1R, the latter functioning like an antibody to react with and block the activity of secreted $TNF\alpha$. These interventions substantially diminish neutrophil accumulation in lungs containing immune complexes, and, accordingly, reduce the intensity of lung injury.

ROLE OF β_2 INTEGRINS

Neutrophil recruitment into rat lungs containing IgG immune complexes has a complicated pattern of requirement for the β_2 integrins, CD11a/CD18 (LFA-1) and CD11b/CD18 (Mac-1). The known counter-receptors for these integrins are ICAM-1, 2 and 3. Another counter-receptor includes the complement activation product, iC3b,

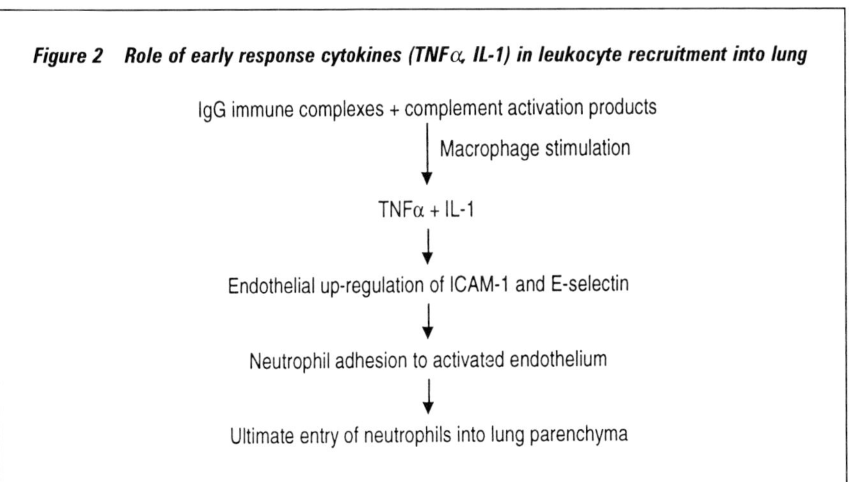

which binds with Mac-1. In the IgG immune complex model, blockade of LFA-1 with intravenous antibody to CD11a substantially reduces neutrophil influx and accompanying tissue damage (Figure 3)[6]. A similar result can be obtained by the intravascular infusion of anti-ICAM 1. Intravenous infusion of blocking antibody to CD11b has no effect in this reaction and fails to reduce neutrophil influx. It appears likely that immune complexes and complement activation products cause lung vascular endothelial up-regulation of ICAM-1 (and E-selectin), facilitating neutrophil adhesion to endothelial ICAM-1. Another important mechanism that leads to neutrophil activation upon contact with the stimulated endothelium is the generation of platelet activating factor (PAF) and IL-8 (or its homologue in the rat) by activated endothelial cells. Both of these are expressed on the surface of the endothelium and can activate adherent neutrophils[7]. It seems likely that this activation process results in a priming of adherent neutrophils such that, upon their transmigration into the alveolar compartment, neutrophils are hyper-responsive to agonists in that area (e.g. cytokines, immune complexes, complement activation products).

A different picture regarding the role of Mac-1 in this inflammatory lung model has emerged (Figure 4). As stated above, when given intravenously, blocking antibody to CD11b was non-protective in the inflammatory model. In striking contrast, intratracheal instillation of anti-CD11b was highly protective in this lung model, whereas similar instillation of anti-CD11a was without effect[6]. These data strongly suggest that the β2 integrin requirements are compartmentalized in the lung, CD11a being linked to intravascular recruitment of neutrophils and CD11b being linked to activation of alveolar macrophages. When anti-CD11b was instilled into the airway, its dramatic protective effects were associated with a substantial fall in the amount of measurable TNFα in bronchoalveolar lavage (BAL) fluids. Airway instillation of anti-ICAM-1 also caused substantial reductions in BAL levels of TNFα and high levels of protection against inflammatory injury. Putting all of these observations together, it appears that alveolar macrophages are tethered to alveolar epithelial cells

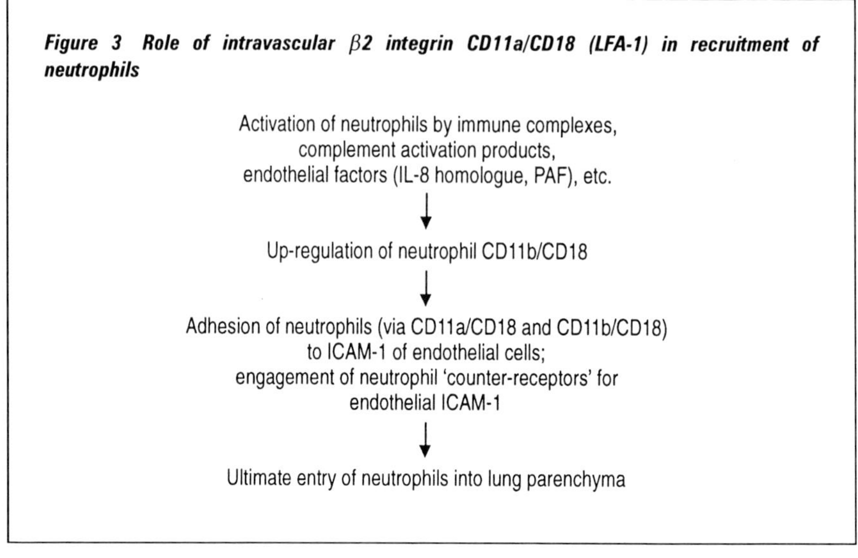

Figure 3   Role of intravascular β2 integrin CD11a/CD18 (LFA-1) in recruitment of neutrophils

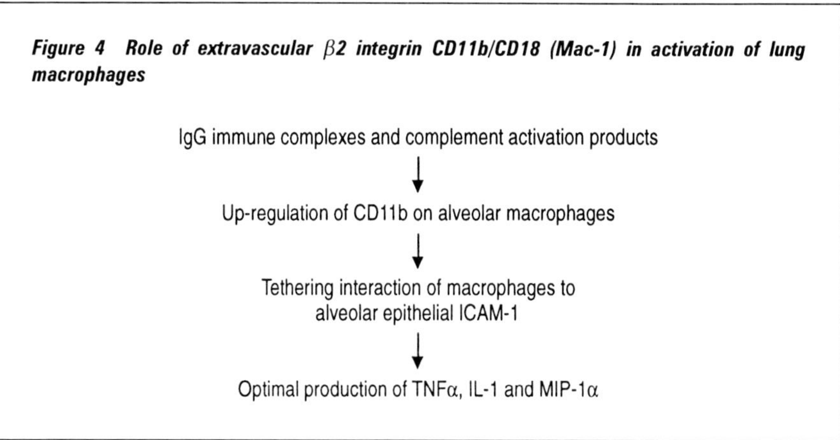

Figure 4   Role of extravascular β2 integrin CD11b/CD18 (Mac-1) in activation of lung macrophages

via CD11b (and CD18) on macrophages and ICAM-1 on epithelial cells. This adhesive interaction, in turn, permits optimal effector function of alveolar macrophages when contact is made with IgG immune complexes and complement activation products. These optimized effector functions probably include cytokine production and oxidant generation by macrophages, both products being linked to development of lung injury involving vascular endothelial cells, alveolar epithelial cells and connective tissue matrix.

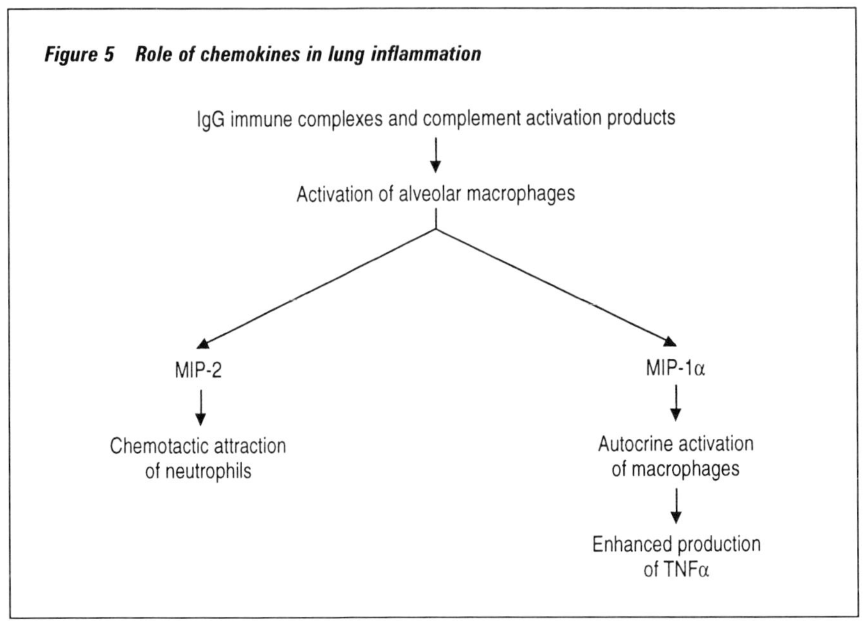

ROLE OF CHEMOKINES

Intrapulmonary deposition of IgG immune complexes results in the activation of lung macrophages to produce at least two different chemokines, cytokines of the IL-8 family. The first chemokine is MIP-2, a C-X-C chemokine with chemotactic and activating properties for neutrophils. Rat MIP-2 has been cloned and reagents for its in vivo blockade developed. mRNA for MIP-2 is detectable within 2 h of immune complex deposition in the lung peaking by 4 h and a gradual decline thereafter. The levels of MIP-2 protein, as determined by ELISA assay, demonstrate a rather similar profile. Most importantly, in vivo blockade of MIP-2 with antibody results in a significant decrease in the numbers of neutrophils accumulating within the alveolar compartment[8] (Figure 5). There is no associated reduction in TNFα levels, suggesting that the role of MIP-2 may be limited to chemotactic function, facilitating the influx of neutrophils adherent to the activated vascular endothelium. In this experimental model MIP-2 appears to be the predominant chemotactic activity recoverable in the BAL fluids (L. Schmid and P A Ward, personal communication).

A second chemokine involved in these inflammatory reactions is MIP-1α, a C-C chemokine with chemotactic and activating activities for T cells and monocytes. As with MIP-2 expression, mRNA for MIP-1α peaks between 2 and 4 h and then dwindles, with a similar pattern for protein expression. In vivo blockade of MIP-1α results in a significant reduction in tissue injury, accompanied by reduced neutrophil influxes[9]. The most unexpected aspect of these findings was the substantial reduction in BAL levels of TNFα in animals in which MIP-1α was blocked. This has led to the

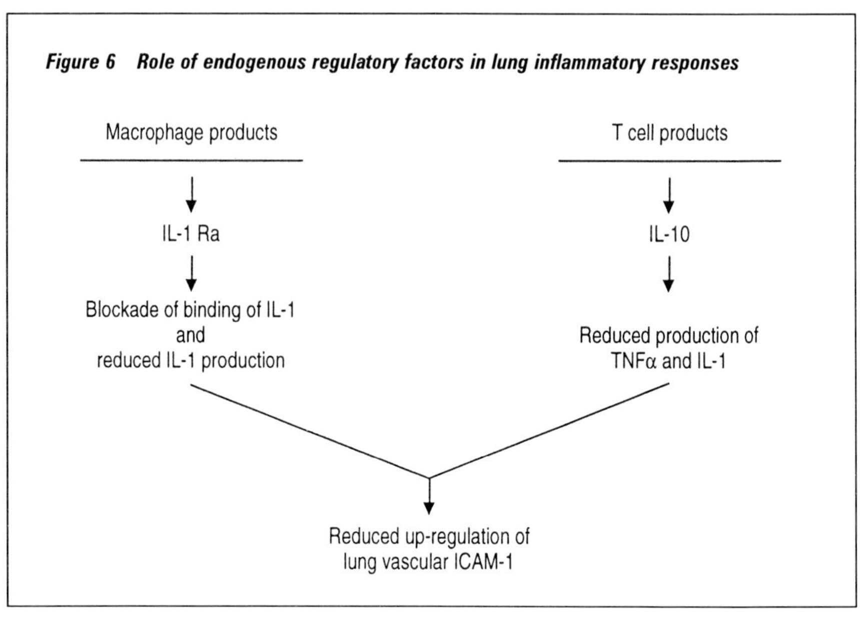

Figure 6   Role of endogenous regulatory factors in lung inflammatory responses

speculation that a major role of MIP-1α is autocrine activation, with a positive feedback loop to macrophages, causing enhanced levels of TNFα, thereby increasing expression of lung vascular ICAM-1. To date, the evidence suggests that RANTES, another C-C chemokine, plays no role in this inflammatory model (T.P. Shanley and P.A. Ward, unpublished observations).

ENDOGENOUS REGULATION OF LUNG INFLAMMATORY RESPONSES

It has been known for some time that the immune complex inflammatory lung model is regulated with respect to duration of the inflammatory response, accumulation of neutrophils, and extent of injury. Specifically, no further haemorrhage and permeability increases occur beyond 4h and there is no further increase in MPO levels in the lung. This suggests that some type of autoregulatory pathway exists in this model of lung injury. Two 'regulatory cytokines' have been identified as playing a role in these inflammatory reactions (Figure 6). Both have been cloned in the rat and reagents developed for in vivo blockade. The IL-1 receptor antagonist (IL-1Ra) has been found in BAL fluids of rats undergoing immune complex deposition in lungs. The protein also peaks at approximately 4h and then diminishes. A similar mRNA pattern has been found. In vivo blockade of IL-1Ra has demonstrated substantial intensification of injury at 4h as reflected by increased permeability values, and a significant increase in numbers of neutrophils recruited into the lung. In vivo blockade of IL-1Ra has been associated with specific increases in BAL content of IL-1 but no significant increase in levels of TNFα[10]. Since IL-1Ra is a known product of activated macrophages, with production peaking after appearance of TNFα and

IL-1, it is an obvious candidate as an endogenous regulator of inflammation. Immunostaining techniques have suggested in the animal model that IL-1Ra is probably contributed both by neutrophils as well as by alveolar macrophages. Precisely why its in vivo blockade leads to a specific increase in IL-1 but not in TNFα remains to be determined.

A second regulatory cytokine involved in these inflammatory responses is IL-10. IL-10 is present in whole lung of rat in significant amounts but after immune complex deposition it is significantly up-regulated, both with respect to mRNA and protein. In animals in which IL-10 has been blocked by the infusion of antibody, there were significant increases in BAL levels of both TNFα and IL-1[11]. This has been associated with increased neutrophil recruitment and intensified injury. These data would strongly suggest that endogenous IL-1Ra and IL-10 play important regulatory roles in diminishing the intensity of injury, ultimately affecting early response cytokine production and, accordingly, expression of endothelial ICAM-1 and E-selectin.

CONCLUSION

Use of the IgG immune complex model of acute inflammatory lung injury in rats has provided useful insights into mechanisms that may be involved in human inflammatory diseases associated with immune complex deposition. This experimental inflammatory model demonstrates an important role for cytokines (TNFα, IL-1) which cause up-regulation of critical adhesion molecules on the activated endothelium. Other cytokines, namely the chemokine (IL-8) family, function both as autocrine stimulators of macrophages (MIP-1α) as well as chemotactic factors (MIP-2). Finally, other products of the cytokine system (IL-1Ra, IL-10) function to suppress the inflammatory response. This information may have important relevance to human inflammatory diseases and their treatment.

Acknowledgements

NIH Grant Support: GM-29507, HL-31963. The author would like to thank Robin Kunkel and Beverly Schumann for their assistance in the preparation of the manuscript.

References

1. Warner RL, Paine R III, Christensen PJ et al. Lung sources and cytokine requirements for in vivo expression of inducible nitric oxide synthase. Am J Resp Cell Mol Biol. 1995;12:649–61.
2. Mulligan MS, Hevel JM, Marletta MA, Ward PA. Tissue injury caused by deposition of immune complexes is L arginine dependent. Proc Natl Acad Sci USA. 1991;88:6338–42.
3. Mulligan MS, Desrochers PE, Chennaiyan AM, Gibbs DF, Johnson KJ, Weiss SJ. In vivo suppression of immune complex-induced alveolitis by secretory leukoproteinase inhibitor and tissue inhibitor of metalloproteinase-2. Proc Natl Acad Sci USA. 1993;90:11523–7.
4. Warren JS, Yabroff KR, Remick DG et al. Tumor necrosis factor participates in the pathogenesis of acute immune complex alveolitis in the rat. J Clin Invest. 1989;84:1873–82.
5. Mulligan MS, Vaporciyan AA, Miyasaka M, Tamatani T, Ward PA. Tumor necrosis factor a regulates in vivo intrapulmonary expression of ICAM 1. Am J Pathol. 1993;142:1739–49.

6. Mulligan MS, Vaporciyan AA, Warner RL et al. Compartmentalized roles for leukocytic adhesion molecules in lung inflammatory injury. J Immunol. 1995;154:1350–63.
7. Zimmerman GA, Prescott SM, McIntyre TM. Endothelial cell interactions with granulocytes: tethering and signaling molecules. Immunol Today. 1992;13:93–100.
8. Schmal H, Shanley TP, Jones ML, Friedl HP, Ward PA. Role for macrophage inflammatory protein-2 in lipopolysaccharide-induced lung injury in rats. J Immunol. 1996;156:1963–72.
9. Shanley TP, Schmal H, Friedl HP, Jones ML, Ward PA. Role of macrophage inflammatory protein-1α (MIP-1α) in acute lung injury in rats. J Immunol. 1995;154:4793–802.
10. Shanley TP, Schrier D, Kapur V, Kehoe M, Musser JM, Ward PA. Streptococcal cysteine protease augments lung injury induced by products of Group A Streptococci. Infect Immun. 1996;64:870–7.
11. Shanley TP, Schmal H, Friedl HP, Jones ML, Ward PA. Regulatory effects of intrinsic IL-10 in IgG immune complex-induced lung injury. J Immunol. 1995;154:3454–60.

16 Adhesion molecules as targets for therapy in rheumatoid arthritis

P. E. LIPSKY, A. F. KAVANAUGH, H. SCHULZE-KOOPS and L. S. DAVIS

Rheumatoid arthritis (RA) is a chronic inflammatory disease, characterized by the entry of mononuclear cells into the synovial tissue and fluid. Activation of these cells initiates the pathogenic events characteristic of the disease[1]. Since the processes that control the entry and accumulation of mononuclear cells in the tissues are critical for the perpetuation of the inflammation, inhibition of recruitment of mononuclear cells into the tissue may attenuate the inflammatory manifestations of RA. It has become evident that physical interactions between the endothelial cells of post-capillary venules and mononuclear cells in the circulation, mediated by a variety of adhesion molecules, govern the entry of inflammatory cells into the tissues[2,3]. Interference with these interactions, therefore, might be effective in the therapy of RA.

The impact of blocking adhesion receptors has been established in animal models of human inflammatory diseases, including those resembling RA[4,5]. Given the key role played by T cells in RA[1,6], one possible target for adhesion receptor directed therapy in this disease would be the adhesion receptor/counter-receptor pair, leucocyte function associated antigen-1 (LFA-1, CD11a/CD18) and intercellular adhesion molecule-1 (ICAM-1, CD54). The interaction of these receptors is critical for trans-endothelial migration of T cells and their subsequent activation[7-9]. By blocking the interaction of LFA-1 with ICAM-1, it might be possible to block migration of T cells into the synovium and their stimulation by locally expressed antigenic peptides in vivo. As a result, amelioration of the signs and symptoms of RA might be anticipated.

To test this hypothesis, a group of patients were treated with a monoclonal antibody (mAb) to ICAM-1[10]. This phase I, dose-escalating study was of open-label design. The primary objectives were to evaluate safety, biological impact and pharmacokinetics, with efficacy as a secondary endpoint. The data, however, are consistent with the conclusion that ICAM-1 plays a central role in rheumatoid inflammation and is, therefore, an important target in the treatment of RA.

METHODS

The initial study population consisted of patients with long-standing RA who met American College of Rheumatology criteria for the diagnosis[11]. To be eligible for enrolment, patients were required to have had disease duration of 4 or more years, and to have failed therapeutic trials with at least two disease modifying anti-rheumatic drugs

(DMARDs). These patients, therefore, had refractory disease. A second trial examined patients with earlier disease who had received no more than one DMARD previously.

The anti-ICAM-1 employed, BIRR-1 (Enlimomab), was of murine origin, and synthesized at Boehringer Ingelheim Pharmaceuticals, Inc. This mAb was an IgG_{2a} mAb, directed against extracellular domain 2 of ICAM-1, which blocks interactions between ICAM-1 and both LFA-1 and MAC-1, another adhesion receptor primarily expressed on neutrophils and monocytes[12]. Blockade of interactions involving the former was considered of greater importance in patients with RA.

For evaluation of clinical efficacy, a modification of the composite criteria established by Paulus et al. was employed[13]. A number of in vitro analyses of immune function of treated patients were carried out as previously described[14,15].

RESULTS

Pharmacokinetics

Initially, it was necessary to assess whether the anti-ICAM-1 mAb could be delivered to achieve a target serum level of $10\,\mu g/ml$, the concentration of mAb that blocks almost all ICAM-1-mediated interactions in vitro[12]. A dose-escalation study was, therefore, carried out in patients, in which varying amounts of mAb were administered over a 5-day period. Dose regimens assessed included total doses of 140 mg (a 60 mg loading dose followed by 4 daily 20 mg doses), 280 mg (a 120 mg loading dose, followed by 4 daily 40 mg doses) and 560 mg (a 240 mg loading dose followed by 4 daily 80 mg doses). Some patients received a total of 240 mg of BIRR-1 over 2 days (120 mg/day). With the intermediate dose of 280 mg, serum antibody levels of up to a mean of approximately $27\,\mu g/ml$ were obtained, and levels throughout the 5-day administration period remained well above the target of $10\,\mu g/ml$; following the 5-day administration period, levels at 8 days were also measurable, but were below $10\,\mu g/ml$. However, by 15 days, mAb was no longer detectable in the serum. The mAb detected in the serum of treated patients was shown to be biologically active as their serum blocked ICAM-1 mediated interactions in vitro, and the degree of blocking correlated with the concentration of ICAM-1 in the serum. These results suggested that a total dose of 280 mg over 5 days would allow the study questions to be addressed, and would be sufficient to estimate whether anti-ICAM-1 has any clinical effects in patients with RA. The adequacy of this dose was confirmed further by examination of synovial fluid from RA patients on the fifth day of administration of anti-ICAM-1, demonstrating the presence of the mAb in the fluid, and hence at the site of inflammation. Immuno-histological evaluation of skin biopsies from treated patients demonstrated that the endothelial cells of the dermis were densely decorated with the anti-ICAM-1. Finally, circulating mononuclear cells were stained to saturation with the mAb[14].

Clinical results

The results obtained with the first 32 refractory patients in this open-label trial were encouraging, demonstrating only mild toxicity and suggesting some therapeutic benefit.

These patients were all treated in a clinical research unit, which could result in a considerable placebo effect. However, nine of these 32 patients received the mAb over a period of only 1 or 2 days and showed minimal clinical benefit. It could, therefore, be argued that the 1- or 2-day treatment group was, in effect, a placebo group, against which the benefit of 5 days of anti-ICAM-1 therapy could be judged.

Of the 23 refractory patients receiving the 5-day protocol, 13 (57%) had a marked or moderate response to treatment from day 8 to day 29 of follow-up. A response was sustained in nine patients up to day 60, and in three up to day 90. The apparent clinical benefits of anti-ICAM-1 were therefore encouraging in this group.

Three of the 10 patients with earlier disease had previously been treated with one DMARD, seven had never received a DMARD and three had only previously been treated with low dose prednisone. The median time from diagnosis was 3 months, although some of the patients had a longer disease duration. All had elevated titres of rheumatoid factor. As has been stressed elsewhere[16], these patients at a relatively early stage, with shorter duration of disease, may represent a more amenable target for intervention than refractory patients with a longer duration of disease.

With the 5-day anti-ICAM-1 treatment protocol, the responses of patients with early disease appeared to be somewhat better than those obtained in the refractory group. Seven of the 10 patients achieved a clinical response up to day 29 of follow-up, and five sustained their response up to day 60. It was particularly noteworthy that three of the patients had long-term clinical benefit, including one patient who met ACR criteria for a complete remission[17] for almost a year after treatment. There were no correlations between the results of treatment and age, gender, or circulating ICAM levels. However, six of the seven patients with early disease who achieved a response at 1 month also manifested decreases of ESR and/or CRP of $\geq 30\%$.

Adverse effects

During therapy, 33 of 42 patients experienced some type of adverse event, but these were mild. Headache, a feature with many mAb therapies, occurred commonly. A number of patients experienced fever or nausea and/or vomiting. Other side effects occurred infrequently. Adverse effects were generally noted on the first or second day of therapy, following which they usually abated, despite continued treatment. They responded to symptomatic treatment, were mild to moderate in terms of severity, and resolved without sequelae. Some of the patients have been followed up for periods of more than 3 years: no infectious complications have been noted. Overall, the anti-ICAM-1 mAb appears to be well-tolerated with no major adverse events noted.

The biological effects of anti-ICAM-1 mAb

Experiments were carried out in order to determine whether particular biological effects of anti-ICAM-1 could be correlated with clinical response. One of the early findings was that the mAb appeared to block the ability of lymphocytes to enter inflammatory sites. This was manifest by the appearance of a peripheral blood lymphocytosis following the first administration of the mAb, that persisted throughout therapy. Thereafter, the levels of circulating lymphocytes returned to normal. There were no significant increases in either neutrophils or monocytes.

Analysis of the phenotype of peripheral blood circulating cells with the fluorescence-activated cell-sorter indicated that, during therapy, there was a significant increase in the numbers of circulating CD3$^+$ T cells. There were no significant changes in circulating B cell numbers. Further analysis revealed that the increase in T cell numbers primarily reflected an increase in CD4$^+$ T cells. Although most of the increase in circulating T cells could be accounted for by CD4$^+$ cells, there was also a small but statistically significant increase in CD8$^+$ T cells during therapy. In the CD4$^+$ population, there was an increase in both memory (CD45RA$^-$) as well as naive (CD45RA$^+$) T cells. In addition, there was an increase in the numbers of activated, circulating T cells, as evidenced by the increased expression of HLA-DR and the α-chain of the IL-2R (CD25). The results are consistent with the conclusion that the T cell lymphocytosis occurred because these cells were blocked from leaving the circulation by the anti-ICAM-1 mAb. This conclusion is supported by the observation that delayed-type hypersensitivity skin testing showed the individuals to be almost uniformly anergic during therapy; 1 month following therapy most of the responses had returned. Biopsy of skin test sites during therapy revealed markedly decreased cellularity, consistent with inhibition of adhesion molecule function.

It seems likely that the administration of anti-ICAM-1 mAb blocked the entry of lymphocytes into inflammatory sites, and presumably into the synovium, and also that it diminished the signs and symptoms of inflammation. In the few patients in whom the delayed type hypersensitivity skin reaction was not blocked by anti-ICAM-1, no clinical response was observed. However, blockade of this reaction could not account wholly for the activity of anti-ICAM-1, since blockade was achieved in most of the remaining patients, but clinical benefit was obtained in only about 60% of cases. In addition, delayed type hypersensitivity was only blocked temporarily, whereas some of the clinical responses extended for 2 months or longer. This raised the question of whether other biological effects of the anti-ICAM-1 might account for the sustained clinical improvement following a short course of treatment. Additional studies in treated patients were carried out to address this possibility. Initial studies examined whether alterations in cytokine patterns might relate to clinical benefit[15]. To investigate this possibility, a reproducible PCR technique to assess cytokine mRNA levels in PBMC was employed that minimized in vitro manipulation of the cells. To determine whether changes in cytokine mRNA levels might be associated with and/or account for the anti-inflammatory effect of anti-ICAM-1 mAb therapy, changes in cytokine mRNA levels were assessed and correlated with clinical improvement. Anti-ICAM-1 mAb administration was followed by a prompt and transient increase in IFN-γ mRNA in peripheral blood mononuclear cells. Elevation of IFN-γ mRNA expression throughout the treatment period reflected the temporary increase in the number of circulating CD3$^+$CD4$^+$ T cells, suggestive of altered circulatory patterns of activated Th1-like T cells, and was related to clinical efficacy. No similar effect on IL-4 mRNA levels in peripheral blood mononuclear cells was observed. The results suggest that anti-ICAM-1 may be beneficial in RA by altering the recruitment of activated Th1-like T cells into the synovium.

A second line of investigation examined whether interference with ICAM-1–LFA-1 mediated interactions might induce a form of peripheral T cell anergy as has previously been described[14]. Analysis of the response of treated patients' T cells demonstrated that long-standing T cell hyporesponsiveness resulted from anti-ICAM-1 treatment. This was associated with a decreased ability of these T cells to produce IL-2, indicating that administration of anti-ICAM-1 had induced typical anergy in these patients. Of importance, the presence of anergy correlated with clinical improvement for prolonged periods of time after the administration of anti-ICAM-1: only one out of the five patients who demonstrated no clinical response developed this form of anergy, whereas anergy was seen in seven of 10 patients who showed a moderate clinical response. All five of the patients with a marked clinical response exhibited anergy at the time clinical outcome was assessed[14]. This suggests that an important aspect of anti-ICAM-1 therapy is the induction of T cell anergy, presumably to synovial antigens, as a result of which sustained clinical response may be obtained. This is not to be confused with the transient cutaneous anergy to irrelevant recall antigens that occurs in most patients, but does not correlate with clinical response and usually returns to normal even though clinical benefit may persist.

DISCUSSION

A novel approach to the treatment of RA has been examined using the adhesion receptor ICAM-1 as a therapeutic target. In animal models of human inflammatory disease, including antigen-induced and adjuvant arthritis models[4,5], blocking LFA-1–ICAM-1-mediated interactions has been shown to abrogate inflammation effectively. Transient inhibition of inflammation would be expected to be beneficial in acute human inflammatory diseases, as is the case in animal models. However, RA is a chronic disease, characterized by persistent inflammation, and presumably driven by the continuous activation of autoreactive T cells[1]. It might be expected that therapy directed against adhesion receptors could effect a long term modulation of the activity of inflammatory disease if additional, more long term effects could be achieved by blocking these interactions. It has been established that adhesion receptors play an important role as accessory molecules in the propagation of immune responses[2,14]. During the generation of immune responses, inhibition of interactions mediated by accessory molecules has been suggested as a mechanism through which immunological tolerance can be induced[16]. Interference with adhesion receptor function might, therefore, induce tolerance to the arthritogenic antigen(s), and thereby achieve long term mitigation of disease activity. Evidence to support this conclusion includes the observation that treatment with anti-LFA-1 and anti-ICAM-1 mAb resulted in long term tolerance to a cardiac allograft in an animal model[18]. Such treatment may also represent an important therapeutic approach to RA.

In the RA patients treated in this study, persistent T cell hyporesponsiveness appeared in some patients after therapy. Importantly, there was a correlation between the generation of this T cell hyporesponsiveness and the induction of a clinical response[14]. This is particularly noteworthy, given the lack of correlation between clinical response and the peripheral lymphocytosis observed during treatment in almost all patients. When circulatory patterns of IFN-γ-producing Th-1-like cells were examined, a clear relationship between trapping these cells in the circulation and clinical benefit was noted[15]. This is consistent with the conclusion that administration of anti-ICAM-1 can block the entry of IFN-γ-producing Th-1-like cells into the synovium and induce anergy of memory cells, presumably responding to synovial antigens, both of which correlate with clinical benefit. The relationship between these two biological effects of anti-ICAM-1 is currently being evaluated.

In summary, administration of anti-ICAM-1 to patients with RA appears to block the entry of Th-1-like IFN-γ-producing cells into inflammatory sites. This action correlates with subsequent clinical benefit. Another important aspect of anti-ICAM-1 therapy in the treatment of RA appears to be the induction of a form of peripheral T cell anergy, largely as a result of which sustained clinical benefit may be obtained.

References

1. Harris ED. Rheumatoid arthritis: pathophysiology and implications for treatment. N Engl J Med. 1990;322:1277–89.
2. Springer TA. Adhesion molecules of the immune system. Nature. 1990;346:425–33.
3. Carlos TM, Harlan JM. Membrane proteins involved in phagocyte adherence to endothelium. Immunol Rev. 1990;114:5–28.
4. Jasin HE, Lightfoot E, Davis LS, Rothlein R, Faanes B, Lipsky PE. Amelioration of antigen-induced arthritis in rabbits treated with monoclonal antibodies to leukocyte adhesion molecules. Arthritis Rheum. 1992;535:541–9.
5. Iigo Y, Takashi T, Tamatani T et al. ICAM-1 dependent pathway is critically involved in the pathogenesis of adjuvant arthritis in rats. J Immunol. 1991;147:4167–71.
6. Strober S, Holoshitz J. Mechanisms of immune injury in rheumatoid arthritis: Evidence for the involvement of T-cells and heat-shock protein. Immunol Rev. 1990;118:233–55.
7. Kavanaugh A, Lightfoot E, Lipsky P, Oppenheimer-Marks N. The role of CD11/CD18 in adhesion and transendothelial migration of T-cells: analysis utilizing CD18 deficient T cell clones. J Immunol. 1991;146:4149–56.
8. Oppenheimer-Marks N, Davis LS, Bogue DT, Ramberg J, Lipsky PE. Differential utilization of ICAM-1 and VCAM-1 during the adhesion and transendothelial migration of human T lymphocytes. J Immunol. 1991;147:2913–21.
9. Wacholtz MC, Patel SS, Lipsky PE. Leukocyte function-associated antigen 1 is an activation molecule for human T cells. J Exp Med. 1989;170:431–48.
10. Kavanaugh AF, Davis LS, Nichols LA et al. Treatment of refractory rheumatoid arthritis with a monoclonal antibody to intercellular adhesion molecule 1. Arthritis Rheum. 1994;37:992–9.
11. Arnett FC, Edworthy SM, Bloch DA et al. The American Rheumatism Association 1987 revised criteria for the classification of rheumatoid arthritis. Arthritis Rheum. 1988;31:315–24.
12. Cosimi AB, Conti D, Delmonico FL et al. In vivo effects of monoclonal antibody to ICAM-1 (CD54) in nonhuman primates with renal allografts. J Immunol. 1990;144:4604–11.
13. Paulus HE, Egger MJ, Ward JR, Williams HJ and the Cooperative Systematic Studies of Rheumatic Diseases Group. Analysis of improvement in individual rheumatoid arthritis patterns treated with disease modifying antirheumatic drugs, based on the findings in patients treated with placebo. Arthritis Rheum. 1990;33:477–89.
14. Davis LS, Kavanaugh AF, Nichols LA, Lipsky PE. Induction of persistent T cell hyporesponsiveness in vivo by monoclonal antibody to ICAM-1 in patients with rheumatoid arthritis. J Immunol. 1995;154:3525–7.
15. Schulze-Koops H, Lipsky PE, Kavanaugh AF, Davis LS. Elevated Th1- or Th0-like cytokine mRNA in peripheral circulation of patients with rheumatoid arthritis: modulation by treatment with anti-ICAM-1 correlates with clinical benefit. J Immunol. 1995;155:5029–37.
16. Waldmann H, Cobbold S. The use of monoclonal antibodies to achieve immunological tolerance. Immunol Today. 1993;14:247–51.
17. Pinal RS, Masi AT, Larsen RA. Preliminary criteria for clinical remission in rheumatoid arthritis. Arthritis Rheum. 1981;24:1308–15.
18. Isobe M, Yagita H, Okumura K, Ihara A. Specific acceptance of cardiac allograft after treatment with antibodies to ICAM-1 and LFA-1. Science. 1992;255:1125–7.

Index